Praise for *Pregnant While Black: Advancing Justice for Maternal Health in America*

"The notorious perils for men in America of 'driving while Black' are well known; the parallel dangers to women in America of driving through a successful pregnancy while Black are far less so. With passion, compassion, and expertise, Monique Rainford exposes and explains this critical disparity, while offering the crucial guidance required to overcome it."

—**David L. Katz**, MD, MPH, past president of the American College of Lifestyle Medicine, and founder and former director of Yale University's Yale-Griffin Prevention Research Center

"Infused with thought-provoking narratives of real maternal-health experiences, this brilliant piece delves into the gut-wrenching facts that contribute to the Black maternal-health crisis across the nation. The strategies and solutions outlined in the text provide one with the insight needed to dismantle maternal-health disparities and inequities."

—**Wanda Irving**, cofounder and chair of the board, Dr. Shalon's Maternal Action Project

"*Pregnant While Black* is the beautiful and profound expansive work on Black maternal health that we've all been waiting for. The book guides us through heartbreaking personal stories using data and evidence to help readers understand the full devastating impact of this very American crisis. Dr. Rainford invites us in to work toward a more equitable and just future for Black pregnant people."

—**Dr. Uché Blackstock**, physician, thought leader on bias and racism in healthcare, and founder of Advancing Health Equity

"In her engaging book, *Pregnant While Black*, the brilliant obstetrician, Dr. Monique Rainford, shows that American Black women of African descent have higher risks of adverse pregnancy outcomes than other women. Her powerful evidence shows that disheartening disparities suffered by Black pregnant women arise not so much from genetic inheritance but more from epigenetic predispositions as the result of generations of racism, inadequate diets, and chronic environmental stress. Nevertheless, Rainford offers encouraging hope for reversing these disparities over the next generation. A must-read for both men and women."

—**Kent Thornburg**, PhD, M. Lowell Edwards Chair of Cardiovascular Research and professor of medicine, Oregon Health & Science University

"Racial disparities still exist in America today, and nowhere is this more apparent than in medicine, where life and death are at stake. Perhaps most tragic are the increased risks seen in young and otherwise healthy pregnant Black women. Black women and their babies die at a higher rate than whites. The reasons underlying these disparities are not clear, nor are they fully explained by classic risk factors such as poverty, education, obesity, or substance abuse. This book explores the insidious roots of these disparities and uncovers the systemic causes. Dr. Rainford brings a unique perspective that allows her to see American medicine through several different lenses and in a way that no one else has been able to bring to life. Dr. Rainford is a Black obstetrician and mother who has seen women's health from many sides. She also practiced medicine in Jamaica, a majority Black country, where she was seen as a privileged professional. Her unique perspective allows her to uncover the real roots of health disparities in the United States; we have never fully understood these, but they become obvious after reading *Pregnant While Black*. This is a scholarly work that is factually detailed yet presented through the personal perspective that Dr. Rainford brings to the problem. It a is must-read for anyone interested in eliminating disparities, as medicine serves as a model for all aspects of human existence. Dr. Rainford gives us a clear path forward."

—**Hugh S. Taylor**, MD, Anita O'Keeffe Young Professor and Chair of the Department of Obstetrics, Gynecology and Reproductive Sciences at Yale School of Medicine; chief of obstetrics and gynecology at Yale–New Haven Hospital

"Dr. Monique Rainford brings knowledge, precision, and more than two decades of experience as an OB/GYN to her book *Pregnant While Black*. As a Black woman, she confronts the complicated crisis of maternal mortality in America with compassion, empathy, and heartfelt storytelling."

—**Linda Villarosa**, author of *Under the Skin: The Hidden Toll of Racism on American Lives and on the Health of Our Nation*

"*Pregnant While Black* takes an unflinching look at a problem that's right before our eyes—the inequitable treatment of Black women who become mothers. Dr. Rainford untangles the multiple social, cultural, political, and racial threads that lead to poorer maternal and fetal outcomes in Black women across America, no matter what their educational attainment or economic level. But this is not a book about hand-wringing. Rather, it's a critical step in calling out the problems of systemic racism in maternal healthcare and finding solutions to this deplorable situation. Kudos to Dr. Rainford for leading the way in changing how pregnant Black women are treated by doctors, healthcare professionals, hospitals, and their community."

—**Neal Baer**, MD, lecturer in global health and social medicine, Harvard Medical School; lecturer in chronic disease epidemiology, Yale School of Public Health; showrunner and executive producer, Netflix

Pregnant
While Black

Pregnant While Black

Advancing Justice for Maternal Health in America

Monique Rainford, MD

Broadleaf Books
Minneapolis

Contents

List of Abbreviations

ACE   adverse childhood experience

ACOG   American College of Obstetricians and Gynecologists

APP   advance-practice practitioner

BMI   body mass index

CDC   Centers for Disease Control and Prevention (US)

CMQCC   California Maternal Quality Care Collaboration

DMV   DC, Maryland, and Virginia

EMR   Electronic Medical Record

FQHC   federally qualified health center

GDM   gestational diabetes mellitus

GPA   Grade point average

HEAL   Health Equity Achieved through Lifestyle Medicine (initiative of the American College of Lifestyle Medicine)

HELLP   hemolysis, elevated liver enzymes, and low platelet count

HMO   health maintenance organization

IAT   Implicit Association Test

IUGR   intrauterine growth restriction

IVF   in-vitro fertilization

KFF   Kaiser Family Foundation

LBW   low birthweight

MBLW   moderately low birthweight

MMRC	maternal mortality review committees
MSDS	Mediterranean-style diet score
NGO	non-governmental organization
NH	non-Hispanic
NHSC	National Health Service Corps
NICU	neonatal intensive care unit
NIH	National Institutes of Health
NIS	Nationwide Inpatient Sample
OB/GYN	obstetrician-gynecologist
PDSA	Plan, Do, Study, Act
SCD	sickle cell disease
SIDS	sudden infant death syndrome
SLE	Significant life event
SMM	severe maternal morbidity
SSA	Sub-Saharan Africa
TDAP	tetanus, diphtheria, and pertussis
VBAC	vaginal birth after cesarean section
VLBW	very low birthweight
WHO	World Health Organization
WIC	Special Supplemental Nutrition Program for Women, Infants, and Children

Prelude

She was about eighteen years old and pregnant with her first child. She was an African American female. She was overweight: technically she would be called obese. She came in because at almost 9 months pregnant she was not feeling her baby move. She was admitted and placed on the fetal monitor. The nurse was unable to find fetal heart tones, and an ultrasound confirmed that the baby was dead. I had never met her before that night. I broke the news to her and her boyfriend, possibly the same age as her. We started the process of inducing labor.

A few hours later, I got a frantic call from one of the nurses. I rushed back to the patient's bedside. My patient was not breathing. We called a code and got all the support we could, but it was already too late. She was dead, and I knew that at least that day there was nothing we could have done to save her life. She likely had an amniotic fluid embolus, a rare pregnancy complication that at that time was thought to be fatal more than 80% of the time.[1] I had to tell that young African American man, still a boy perhaps, that he not only lost the baby that he was looking forward to fathering but one of the loves of his short life.

Now, almost two decades later, I wonder if the healthcare system could have saved her. Not that night, because I know there was nothing else we could have done, but could we have done more to prevent the events that led to the death of her baby and increased her own risk, which ultimately led to her death? What could we as physicians have done? What could we in healthcare have done?

Introduction

Black women in America are three times more likely to die from pregnancy than if they are described as White. Race as a risk factor has nothing to do with the woman's genetic code and too much to do with the social systems in America—systems that have been in place for decades and that are not being dismantled quickly enough. Structural racism—the systems and policies which reinforce racial inequities—increase a Black woman's likelihood of having more life-threatening complications but also increase her likelihood of receiving suboptimal care for these complications. Racism in its many forms makes it more dangerous for a Black woman to have her baby in the United States of America, where her risk of dying from a pregnancy-related complication during pregnancy or in the first 42 days after pregnancy was more than 40 in 100,000 even before the Covid-19 pandemic. By comparison, during that period the risk for a Mexican woman having her baby in Mexico was 33 in 100,000, and 25 in 100,000 for a Grenadian woman having her baby in the small Caribbean Island of Grenada.

Black mothers across socioeconomic classes are needlessly dying, and as a practicing Black obstetrician and gynecologist, I have learned that education and class do not protect us nor do they lessen our maternal death rate.

Is this a new problem? The answer is no. But, what is new is that within the past seven years this issue has made it to mainstream media due to the work of several investigative journalists, including the groundbreaking work of Nina Martin, who tracked and identified 134 of the 700–900 women who died from pregnancy-related causes in 2016,[1] and published some of their heart-wrenching stories in *ProPublica* and on NPR, as well as the continuing outstanding and impactful work of Linda Villarosa, who has spent decades exposing the health inequities that affect Black people in America. Another reason is the selfless advocacy work of the women's families, including Charles Johnson, the son of the TV judge Glenda Hatchett, who lost his wife Kira Johnson, and Wanda Irving, who lost her daughter Shalon Irving, both due to circumstances that leave many pained and bewildered. Both women were successful, highly educated Black women. In addition, advocates such as Dr. Joia Crear-Perry, the founder and president of the National Birth Equity Collaborative, have used the fuel of their own difficult birth experiences to advocate for change. And celebrities, including Serena Williams and Beyoncé Knowles-Carter, have been talking about their near-death delivery experiences. Finally, a tragedy is being recognized for what it is—not a Black tragedy but an American tragedy—and is receiving well overdue attention.

It was at Harvard Medical School that I first noticed that these disparities existed. I remember sitting in a class in the amphitheater of the conference center, now known as the Joseph B. Martin Conference Center, reading what I considered a startling statistic presented on a slide. The infant mortality rate for Black American babies was worse than that of Jamaican babies and more than double the rate of their White counterparts. I could have easily missed it. It was one of many numbers on a busy slide. However, that statistic, which I still remember some thirty years later, had a significant impact on me. While, on the one hand, I was pleased that Jamaica had relatively good statistics for a developing country, I could not understand how this first-world country, with all its modern facilities, could have such trouble caring for its citizens. If there was a substantive discussion about it at the time, I certainly do not recall. I suspect there was not.

Over the years I often heard the same answers: the disparity was the result of socioeconomic factors. It was not until many years later that I learned that the disparity in health between Black women and White women remains even when socioeconomic factors are accounted for. Poverty could never have told the entire story because poverty was definitely a factor in Jamaica too. I heard other explanations, which were unsatisfactory. However, being swept up in the demands of medical school and residency, I left it there.

Years later, after I returned to Jamaica and set up a gynecology and obstetrics practice, and then came back to live in the United States in 2014, I would come to a better understanding of the real factors that contributed to the disparities: racism in its many forms and its consequences. I listened to two TED talks, which discussed the effect of racism on the health of African Americans. The first was by Miriam Zoila Perez where she talked about the JJ way[2]—a model of delivering prenatal care established by Jennie Joseph, a British-trained midwife; then Dr. David Williams discussed how racism was making Black men in America sick.[3] It was an "aha" moment for me because finally there was another piece of the puzzle, perhaps the most important piece. It was not necessarily about direct acts of racism but sometimes-subtle, unconscious or implicit bias, such as not giving the patient as much medical attention as she deserves due to her race—frankly, giving her substandard care—or making race-based assumptions about her. It is about social structures that have been in place for years that continue to discriminate against African Americans. It was the way an African American pregnant woman might be treated on a day-to-day basis. Unfortunately, I have observed this implicit bias in professional settings throughout my career, but, having been raised in Jamaica, I did not always recognize it for what it was at the time. It was a feeling that something was not quite right, but I did not yet have the words or the knowledge to understand what was wrong.

Trying to understand the idea of structural racism and implicit bias and its impact on the care Black women received meant looking back at my own experience as a Black woman in America. I was born in Brooklyn, New York, to Jamaican immigrants. Facing the racism that still existed in New York at the time of my birth in the 1970s, my father wanted a better life for his family. He was certain that remaining in America at that time would have thwarted his professional growth and stifled the opportunities he was able to provide for his family. My mother, having just completed a Master of Arts in Nutrition from New York University within six months of my birth, was open to the possibilities, including her husband's desire to return to their homeland. So it was that my two-year-old brother and I, an eleven-month-old baby, flew home to Jamaica with my parents. My pride and keen awareness of my dual citizenship was manifested in different ways; in my elementary school career I promptly stood up in my second grade class when my teacher asked if there was anyone from another country in the class, my off-key belting of the star-spangled banner and attempt to play it on the piano in the living room of my house in Kingston, Jamaica, and the certainty I had at age ten that I was not only going to pursue tertiary education in the United States but that I would be attending Harvard.

I thrived in Jamaica. I was at the top of my class from kindergarten B to fourth grade. At the end of grade 4, I took and passed a special entrance exam and earned a seventh-grade place in one of Jamaica's top high schools for girls, Immaculate Conception High. The fact that the transition was easy speaks of the excellent preparation I had in elementary school. At the end of my first year, at the age of eleven, I proudly walked on the stage at the year-end prize-giving ceremony multiple times having achieved first place in multiple subjects in the entire seventh grade of more than 200 students.

However, to say I was an all-rounder at the time would be a stretch. I was a subpar athlete at best; was informed by my always-loving but equally blunt mother at age 7 that I could not sing (hence my decision to abandon my career goal as a singer); and was decidedly socially awkward. I may have won awards as a scholarly nerd but would not have made the cool girls' list.

My initial decision to become a doctor occurred at the age of seven. My chin split open when my brother and I were jumping from the bed, an activity we both knew we should never do. I was carefully bandaged, but my caregiver at the time opted not to disturb my parents at work. Hours later when they arrived, they were shocked to find the state of their only girl. We immediately went to Oxford Medical Center, what would have been the equivalent of an urgent care at that time. I was carefully sutured by the physician working that evening. He was a kind, compassionate, slightly overweight dark-skinned gentleman of medium height. He rewarded me for my bravery with a fifty-cent coin. He became a hero in my seven-year old's eyes, and I immediately knew I wanted to be like him when I grew up.

High school at Immaculate was intellectually exciting. I was exposed to a variety of subject areas, including some of my favorites in the earlier years: Latin, history, chemistry, and Spanish. Maybe I could be a translator or a lawyer, I thought.

Then tragedy struck. Word reached my parents that my elementary-school principal was in the hospital. I loved Sister Pat. I remember her attentively listening to me sing and deciding to allow me a place in the choir—a position, I realized later, was largely based on my strong enthusiasm to sing rather than my raw talent. I remember her choosing me and a fellow classmate to represent Mary and Joseph for a school assembly, but quickly realizing that it was overwhelming for the somewhat shy first-grader who had a secret crush on the would-be Joseph. My parents took me to the hospital, and I went into her room. She was lying in bed in a cotton night gown, her flowing hair no longer covered by her veil. Always being a thin woman, she appeared slight, as her freckled olive-brown face rested on her pillow. Her attentive administrative assistant was by her side. Sister Pat shared with my thirteen-year-old self her heartfelt desire, "I wish I had more time." At barely forty years old, her time on this earth was about to be over. My calling to be a doctor was cemented, but my role was less clear. I thought I wanted to be a pediatrician who also worked on finding the cure for cancer.

Four years later, despite my father's reluctance to let his baby girl go, I embarked on the plane to America with my parents to take up my freshman position at the University of Pennsylvania. I thought I knew a lot about America. After all, I had spent several enjoyable and exciting summers with my cousins in New York. I knew you could get whatever you wanted at the stores. I felt I had arrived, when, as a teenager, I had a temp job in the city and took the subway with busy New York professionals to Chinatown, picked up my delicious bagel with cream cheese at the food truck, and joined the rat race at my job. I watched almost exclusively American TV, which was readily available in Jamaica and was certain I wanted to be one of the cool sorority girls I had watched in all those movies.

However, when I arrived at the University of Pennsylvania, I saw something different. While the distinction of what it meant to be White or Black in America did not occur to me as I watched TV, it was very real to me after a short stay at the university. Perhaps the reality was that growing up in Jamaica I did not see being Black as being different. I was not a "minority" in Jamaica, a majority Black country; I was never asked to check a category marked "Black." There were no negative racial connotations associated with who I was. I was a child with privilege—two professional parents, a father who often talked of his humble beginnings. My father, one of nine children, grew up with his widowed mother and, shoeless, attended school in his early days in a hilly, rural community in St. Catherine, Jamaica, and worked his way up to owning a large five-bedroom house on the slopes of one of Jamaica's most sought-after neighborhoods.

It did not fully occur to me that all the sorority girls I identified with and wanted to emulate were White, and apart from the late great Whitney Houston there were very few, if any, Black girls or women on American TV in the 1980s whom I felt I wanted to emulate. Furthermore, I now realize that I, too, was subject to the brainwashing by American media at the time to believe that there was something inherently wrong with African Americans, but that this certainly did not include my singing idols like Whitney Houston or Prince.

At Penn, I quickly became aware of the distinct color lines dividing an American university, where people of largely the same race sat together. In the cafeteria, there was the Black table, the White table, the Asian table. I sought desperately to reject the notion and to find where I fit in, but it was difficult. I was Black but not African American, and as such, while I participated in a number of activities during my undergrad years, including multiple-step shows from the proud Black fraternities and a fantastic fashion show where I proudly modeled African garments with a handsome African American upper classman, I knew I did not fit in. I spent time in the Caribbean community, and, though meaningful, it was too small to sustain my sense of belonging.

It was not until my second year when I felt a stronger sense that I had established a community. I decided to serve as a residential advisor in one of the less-cool dorms at Penn where I had lived my first year. My closest friends were a Japanese American who grew up in the suburbs of Philadelphia and a Caribbean American who grew up in the Bronx, New York, ironically only a few blocks from the cousins I had spent so many summers visiting. Our larger group consisted of a tall Korean American, a short chubby Jewish American, and a slightly taller, but by no means tall, Southeast Asian American. I felt we were the misfits, the non-cool kids, but we formed a social life with one another that made college life much more enjoyable.

Something else happened in those undergraduate years: I began to doubt my right or ability to be at the University of Pennsylvania because of the narrative of affirmative action that several people shared with me. Making the Dean's List as a chemistry major during my first year at college did little to dispel the myth that I was not qualified to be there but only got the place because I was Black. Having broken my leg in my second year of university and taking a physical chemistry course that I found particularly difficult, which led to a downward shift in my GPA, did little to strengthen my confidence.

Even my acceptance to multiple medical schools, in addition to Harvard, the one I chose, did not strengthen my confidence.

However, Harvard Medical School restored my hope in the American dream. I was pre-med from the beginning of Penn and leapt at the opportunity to graduate in three years and accept my place at Harvard Medical School. My childhood dreams were falling into place. After graduating from Penn, I arrived at a large, welcoming medical-school environment. One of my White classmates also vocally expressed his amazement at being accepted to Harvard Medical School. However, he admitted something I would never dare to admit, his GPA. It was comparable to mine, and I finally realized that I had earned my place and I was certainly no less qualified than any other student there. Another classmate, this time Southeast Asian, offered another welcome—which to him was a small gesture. When I shared it with him recently, he did not recall it, but to me it was a huge thing. I was lamenting with a small group of Black students my disappointment with the seeming lack of integration in American society. They, despite having immigrant parents, had spent much of their formative years in this country and they felt that "how it is" was a given at the time. However, as I walked outside Vanderbilt Hall, the Southeast Asian student asked me if I would like to join fellow classmates in a game of tag football in the quad, the open area of grass surrounded on three sides by imposing Harvard buildings. I remember nothing of the game because I have little interest in American football, but I never forgot the gesture. America was and remains to me the land of opportunity for people from multiple cultures, races, and ethnicities, and the best of this country to me is an environment where there is an embrace of these cultures. That is how I felt at Harvard Medical School. My participation in the Black student organization was not seen as being separate but was embraced by the larger community, and my closest friends from medical school, in addition to strong connections with my fellow Black students, ultimately consisted of a multicultural group of individuals with Asian, Anglo, Jewish, and Latino backgrounds. I also found strong social support in the Jamaican university community in Cambridge.

However, I was still scarred by the culture shock of what it felt like to be Black in America. I experienced an overt racist verbal attack early in my undergraduate years, and it took me only a few months after arriving at Penn to decide that I wanted to return to Jamaica to spend the rest of my life. The planner that I was, it would have to be after I completed all my education and paid down a significant portion of my debt.

One night, while returning with my friend from a party, a vehicle with three young White men pulled near to us. We were already on the Penn campus, only a few yards from our dorm. One young man leaned through the window and asked, "How much?"

My girlfriend, a fearless Caribbean American from New York, promptly told them off. I remember one of the men saying the only thing good you have is the white teeth. Interestingly, although I remember it more than thirty years later, my friend has no recollection of the event. She chalks it down to having so many similar lived experiences. My desire to return to Jamaica, although partly due to the bond I had with my family, was not fueled by opportunities that existed there but rather by the certainty that having to endure such experiences would be harmful to me psychologically. I had no idea at that time how much more harmful it could be, and was, for Black people across America.

During medical school, I deviated from my almost-certain plan of pursuing pediatrics. Perhaps not ironically, I shifted my path because of a powerful birthing experience. In my third year of medical school, the Vice-Chairman of Obstetrics and Gynecology at the Beth Israel Hospital, Dr. Henry Klapholz, allowed me to assist with a delivery. The love and tears of joy that poured out from the new parents, a French couple, are forever seared into my memory. I did not fully realize it at that time, but my fate was sealed. I would commit to a career as a physician in the field of obstetrics and gynecology and would remain committed to women's health.

After completing a residency program in Washington, DC, where I had the privilege of serving patients from all walks of life, I went on to choose jobs that initially focused on the care of the underserved, whether economically disadvantaged Black or White Americans,

Latinos, other people of color, or immigrants. While the institutions I worked with ensured that people had access to healthcare, and while in some cases surgical services were limited, I felt that the obstetric care that we offered had all the first-world advantages. I remember caring for an African American woman with HIV in the early 2000s. She did well during her first pregnancy but had a subsequent pregnancy in short order. At a time when treatment options were far less advanced than they are today and the patient's prognosis was grimmer, I was convinced that she would not make it, but was relieved when I saw her months later, still during her pregnancy, with improved medications that made her look healthy again. I remember having attended, during my training, to an African American woman with a serious bleeding complication due to a condition called placenta previa, in which the placenta covers the opening of the cervix at the time of childbirth. She spent several hours in the operating room, while my senior colleague and our supervising physicians tried to stop her bleeding. Her life hung in the balance. Later, when I attended to her while she was recuperating in the ICU, I was not sure she would make it because she had lost her full blood volume many times over and received in excess of fifteen units of blood. But she made a full recovery. Also important, although I did not recognize how important at the time, she was cared for by a team with multiple Black doctors.

In both cases, the mothers survived partly because of the resources available here, in the US hospitals I worked in. In many countries outside the United States, the abundance of blood products or life-saving HIV medications would not be available. The state-of-the-art ICU care would sometimes be impossible. However, there was another component that was key—something that never dawned on me as being significant at the time. Their healthcare team included many Black physicians and nurses.

But I also remember instances of disparities that I noticed during my training and being told it was due to poverty or the insinuation that such an outcome was expected. One patient comes vividly to my mind. I think of her often. I think of her when I am informed of any possibility that healthcare for women could be compromised. I think of her when I encourage women to have Pap smears. I think of her when I examine the health disparities experienced by African American women.

I call her Jenny. Jenny was a thirty-three-year-old African American woman whom I cared for during my residency training. She was only a few years older than I was at the time, but she was dying from cervical cancer, a cancer that is almost 100% preventable by timely Pap screening. But Jenny's suffering was not just about the pain that we often hear being experienced by people with end-stage cancer. It was something that had a more profound effect on her womanhood. Jenny's cancer, as advanced stage cervical cancer does, had eroded from her cervix through the walls of her vagina through her bladder and rectum. She was incontinent of both urine and stool. It meant that the canal that allows childbirth was no longer separated from the canal designed for waste. She was forced to wear diapers. Despite that Jenny still had a cheerful disposition, and when I visited her, she had a radiant smile, a smile that I will always remember. With what I have learned since, I have so many more questions about why Jenny died of such an advanced case of a cancer that is almost completely preventable in a country that has abundant resources.

Four and a half years after completing my training I returned to Jamaica. My lived experiences between the time I was a naive freshman in college and my career as a high-earning, established obstetrician and gynecologist did little to dissuade me that my experience of being Black in Jamaica was far better than what I experienced in the United States. I was comfortable with sometimes being an "other," but I would never be comfortable with being viewed as "less than," which was something I never experienced in Jamaica. I continued to strive to ensure that the care I delivered to my patients was consistent with the recommendations of the American College of Obstetricians and Gynecologists (ACOG), and made it a priority to deliver equitable care to my patients regardless of their financial situation.

Life definitely does not always go as planned. Nine years after I returned to Jamaica, it struck me that I needed to return to America. My motivation was similar to that of my father's, but my thoughts were different from those he had had so many years before. I was definitely concerned about racism and race in America and how it would impact my two children. But, ultimately, my husband and I decided— or hoped—that the financial opportunities that we would personally be able to offer them if we continued our careers in the United States would exceed those available in Jamaica. It was no longer only about my wants. I now had to think about the financial legacy I would leave to my children. But I was very mindful of the cost of that legacy, so I worried. Would I be able to protect their self-esteem and confidence while raising them in the United States? However, I had hope: a Black family was in the White House. They had two children like me, and every indication suggested that their daughters were doing well. Perhaps that was a lofty comparison, but we were moving to the Washington, DC, metropolitan area where the first family also lived, and I thought if they could do it, so could we.

When my husband and I decided to return to the United States, things were already changing for me, even before I realized it. My first job selection was a private practice, which served a diverse population, and I did not notice any disparity among my patients, but that is not to say it did not exist. Yet I still remember my young, healthy, economically advantaged African American patient delivering a little before full term. Why? I was confident she was receiving quality care at my practice. She had no obvious risk factors, yet she went into labor prematurely. I did not yet realize that being Black in America was a risk factor that had nothing to do with her economic status or genetic background.

I enjoyed serving this population, but for economic reasons moved on to another job after a year. This time, I was again serving the underserved and economically disadvantaged, including primarily African American, Latino, and immigrant patients from multiple countries. I have always had a sense of pride when I was able to deliver "first-class care" to some of those who would not otherwise get it. However, while I was not necessarily surprised that new immigrants and undocumented persons would not always get access to this care due to lack of insurance, I naively expected that with the Affordable Care Act that was now in place any US citizen could easily acquire insurance and access to quality care, but I was sorely mistaken.

The more I learned about the health disparities for African Americans and other Black people in America, the more I wanted to do something about them and help those with less of anything to have more, a desire likely born from a core value of equity. This desire was shaped by the countless volunteer activities my parents exposed me to while I was growing up. The class disparities were readily apparent in Jamaica, and my parents were committed to helping those economically disadvantaged, my father never forgetting his humble beginnings. My mother, having observed the sacrifices her parents had made to ensure that she and her siblings had a comfortable upbringing, felt that she should do her best to help others enjoy the lifestyle that she had had. I was spurred on as well by the now-certain knowledge that the disparities were due to racism. I had already gained a personal understanding of what it felt like to be treated as "less than," something many, if not all, African Americans have experienced in their life.

The interest led me to comb through the literature so that I could fully understand the nature and the causes of the problems. This led me to discover and tell the story of Dr. Shalon Irving (an African American woman who died 3 weeks after childbirth) in a TEDx talk.[4] It led me to deliver Grand Rounds (a formal meeting in the hospital setting where physicians and other health professionals attend lectures for medical education) on the topic, in the hospitals I was affiliated with in Baltimore and now at Yale. It has led me to actively participate in medical education with the hopes that the future generations of doctors will be better and do better. It continues to drive me to write and speak about the topic. It has led me to become a member of multiple taskforces devoted to anti-racism and promoting diversity, equity, and inclusion. It has led me to write this book.

This book is about more than my research. It encompasses experiences from my twenty-three years of experience as an obstetrician and gynecologist, who has cared for women of multiple races in a variety of settings. It will encompass knowledge I have acquired during my nine years as a member of the American College of Lifestyle Medicine. I will share the stories of friends and colleagues who have had to experience the system as a Black woman and how it failed them. It will delve into my own birthing story and how the decision to return to Jamaica when I did may have been more protective that I could ever fathom. But most importantly it will offer tangible strategies to effect change by carefully detailing programs that have been successful and offering further solutions.

I have written this book to help protect every Black woman who is having a baby in America or desires to have one. It is written for healthcare professionals who care for these women and their babies. It is written for the institutions that train these professionals. It is written for the institutions that deliver the care. It is written for politicians who believe that the value of a woman's life should not be based on the color of her skin. And it is intended for global leaders who want to participate with America in righting its wrongs.

CHAPTER 1

Why Black Mothers Are Dying in America

While I just spent some time describing the journey that led me to write this book, I only superficially mentioned that the root of the disparities in Black maternal health is structural racism and implicit bias, but what does that all mean and how is it so dramatically increasing the maternal health risk of Black women? While many of you who choose to read this book may already know what these terms mean, I know many do not.

Let's start with structural racism. It refers to "the totality of ways in which societies foster racial discrimination through mutually reinforcing systems of housing, education, employment, earnings, benefits, credit, media, healthcare, criminal justice. These patterns and practices in turn reinforce discriminatory beliefs, values and distribution of resources."[1]

While the root of this goes back to slavery, how does it play out in the lives of a pregnant African American woman and by extension any Black woman in America? For the purpose of this book, I will offer a simplified version of the explanation since I readily acknowledge that there are a great number of books and articles that delve into this topic in the detail that it deserves.

I visited the National Museum of African American History and Culture with my late cousin, Michelle, on April 25, 2017. This visit was pivotal in my understanding of the roots of racism in America. It was there I first learned about the social origins of the current definitions of race. Race categorizations were man-made, motivated by power and greed.[2] I learned there was a time in the 1600s when poor White and Black people bonded together in an attempt to improve their situation, but Whites in power squashed the unity by assigning more privilege and authority to the Whites, essentially pitting one group against the other.

Over time, I gained a better understanding of ways that African Americans were constantly being denied upward mobility, even after slavery had been abolished and some of the harsh restrictions placed on them to sabotage advancement continued in the subsequent years. When communities did advance, many were destroyed by their fellow White Americans, likely stoked by hatred built on years of being taught and embracing a belief that their fellow Black Americans were inferior. An outstanding example is the Tulsa Massacre.

Further advancement continued to be limited by racial segregation in schools, the failure of the GI Bill in the equitable assignment of benefits to Black veterans, the prevention of Black home ownership through redlining, to name only a few examples. Unfortunately, modern-day examples of school segregation also exist. Schools in predominately Black areas continue to suffer from poorer performance and funding than schools in predominantly White districts. It helped me to understand why in 2019 the average wealth of a Black family was less than 15% of that of a White family.[3]

How does this oppression extend beyond economics? It also speaks of the excess stressors on African American women even before they get pregnant and throughout their pregnancy. If a society constantly marginalizes you and constantly makes it harder for you to succeed, socially, financially, and professionally, even if you do succeed, it takes a toll on your health. Exactly what type of a toll? This toll is multifactorial.

Let's start with the stressors of yesterday, affecting the parents, grandparents, and great-grandparents of the African American women of today. I first learned about the field of epigenetics from an excellent presentation by Dr. Kent Thornburg at one of the annual conferences of the American College of Lifestyle Medicine.[4] Epigenetics is the study of how behaviors and environment can cause changes that affect the way genes work or are expressed.[5] Changes in how a gene is expressed can be passed from generation to generation without affecting the genetic code. In other words, the problem does not fundamentally lie in normal genetic composition of Black people, but in how certain factors can affect how genes function in the body.

Another term I feel I need to define is "programming." "Programming," as the name suggests, refers to the association between an environmental stress in the womb and the development of a disease in later life. As Dr. Thornburg and his colleague Dr. Wallack eloquently outlined in the research articles,

Vulnerability for chronic and other diseases, both physical and mental, is "programmed" into human biology much earlier than we thought—preconception through the first 1000 days to about age two. Nutrition, is critical, and we now know that impacts of intergenerational disease-generating "toxic" stress caused by interlocking systems of oppression that lead to institutional racism, financial deprivation, lack of opportunity, and limited access to resources resulting in disadvantaged position in society must also be addressed.[6]

Simply put, the effects of slavery, Jim Crow, persistent economic barriers, continued mistreatment of Black people, based on a completely avariciously designed human notion that Black people are lesser human beings, can affect a developing baby in the womb. If this baby is a girl, it further affects the baby girl's developing eggs—the same eggs that can ultimately be mobilized for the conception of her own children. Epigenetic effects may not only affect the birthweight of the baby but lead to increased risk of conditions that Black women disproportionately suffer. For example, if the effects lead to the baby having a low birthweight (weighing less than 2,500g) that child already has an increased risk of hypertension, coronary artery disease, and type 2 diabetes. Babies having an excessively high birthweight (about 5,000g or more), with a diabetic mother, are at an increased risk of obesity and type 2 diabetes and metabolic syndrome.[7] Epigenetic effects can even be present if the baby is normal weight. It does not stop there.

During her college years, Professor Arline Geronimus worked part-time at a school for pregnant teenagers in Trenton, NJ. She noticed that these teenagers were suffering from health conditions that her White and more affluent classmates rarely had.[8] She used the term "weathering" to describe an early deterioration in the health of Black people due to the additive negative effects of repeated experiences of having to face social or economic adversity and being marginalized politically.[9] Building on the work of Geronimus, McEwan and Stellar later defined *allostatic load*, "the wear and tear on the body which accumulates over time after exposure to repeated or chronic stress."[10] Studies have shown that this load was worse for Black women than for White women or even Black men; and for Black people in America, the load was similar to that of White people who were ten years older. Furthermore, non-poor Blacks were more likely to have higher scores than poor Whites, reinforcing the findings that the fact that Black people were found to have excessive rates of higher allostatic loads was not explained by the higher proportion of Black people who were poor.[11] What's the problem with having a higher allostatic load? People with higher allostatic load scores have an increased risk of dying compared to similarly aged people with lower scores,[12] and have an increased risk of having more illnesses, including cardiovascular disease. Studies have even found a link between higher allostatic loads and preeclampsia,[13] a condition I will describe in more detail later in this book.

The impact of the chronic stress of racism on the health of African American women was further quantified by Elizabeth Blackburn. She discovered the molecular nature of telomeres, the protective tips at the ends of chromosomes. Shorter telomeres have been associated with increased incidence of diseases and increased likelihood of dying younger than expected.[14] Working with psychologist Elissa Epel, Blackburn realized that the caregivers (mothers) of children with chronic illnesses had shorter telomeres than expected. Not surprisingly, the longer their time as caregivers, the shorter the length of their telomeres. There was another fascinating finding from the research that I will write about later: The more the mother perceives her situation as being more stressful, the shorter her telomeres. Black women in America, ages 49–55, have been found to have shorter telomeres than White women, suggesting an approximate biological aging of approximately 7.5 years.[15] This suggests that a Black woman has the biological age of a White women who is 7.5 years older than her. This correlates with the work of Professor Geronimus where the difference was ten years.

Black women in America are therefore more likely to have chronic health conditions at younger ages compared to White women in America, further increasing their risk of having these conditions even before they get pregnant, which in itself makes their pregnancy riskier. But that is not all. An adverse event in childhood can lead to an adverse childhood experience (ACE). Studies have shown that individuals with at least four ACEs were at increased risk of health conditions, including overweight and obesity, diabetes, cancer, heart disease, respiratory disease, and mental illness, compared with individuals with no ACEs.[16] Non-Hispanic Black children in America have more ACEs than children of any other race.[17]

It gets more disappointing. Even if a Black woman is college-educated, even if she was able to maintain her health despite the multiple odds against her, she is still more likely to suffer from severe maternal morbidity compared to women of other races who never graduated from high school. This is despite the fact that the rate of severe maternal morbidity tends to be lower for college graduates compared to women who did not graduate from high school.[18]

I have mentioned that the disparities that Black women experience are not related to their actual genetic code. I will provide multiple examples throughout this book where African American women have poorer maternal health and infant outcomes compared to African born mothers or Caribbean born mothers despite shared African ancestry.

Then there is the other side—the side that sheds even more light on why Black pregnant and postpartum women continue to suffer sometimes deadly consequences, even if they try their very best to do everything right for their pregnancy. Implicit bias—or unconscious biases—are biases that individuals have without realizing it. Unfortunately, even clinicians who are called to deliver unbiased care to all their patients have as much implicit bias as everybody else.[19] These biases, which lead to negative assumptions about someone because of their race or other factors, have a negative impact on the delivery of care, including diagnosis, treatments, and the level of care patients receive. Studies have shown that the more pro-White the bias is, the less likely a Black patient will receive the recommended treatment than a White patient.[20] This finding is further compounded by a study which evaluated implicit preference of medical doctors for White Americans compared to Black Americans using the Implicit Association Test (IAT), a well-established measure of implicit bias. Except for African American doctors, all the doctors in the study which also included Asian, Hispanic, and White doctors had an implicit preference for White Americans over Black Americans.[21] Many clinicians, therefore, may be discriminating against their patients without realizing it, while thinking all along that they are giving their patients the very best care, regardless of race. But they are not.

How do individuals develop these negative assumptions against Black people? Even a brief study of American history, which is replete with examples of blatant, subtle, and not-so-subtle attacks on Black people, will reveal multiple answers. No study is needed, however, to confirm that the problem persists. A cursory look at present-day America makes us painfully aware of this. However, there is an additional troubling side to this already disturbing fact: People generally have biases in favor of their own group. European Americans' implicit pro-ingroup bias appears consistent and stable over time. For African Americans, however, this is not so. Half of African Americans have implicit pro-Black over pro-White bias, while the other half reveals an implicit pro-White over pro-Black bias.[22] Was that different in the study with the doctors? Actually no. While, overall, African American doctors did not have a preference for White Americans over Black Americans, when evaluated further, that neutral effect arose because some African American physicians had an implicit preference for White Americans and others had an implicit preference for Black Americans. In other words, albeit to a lesser extent, Black clinicians could be responsible for delivering substandard care to patients of their own race because they did not escape society's negative influence in how they perceive their own race. This certainly includes Black doctors coming from other regions like the Caribbean or the continent of Africa because as I mentioned before, and as embarrassed as I am to admit it, I did not have the most positive opinion of African Americans when I came back to the United States for college. I am just grateful that my eyes were opened.

Fortunately, research has shown that if, as clinicians, we care to be better, and do better, implicit-bias training can improve this negative trend and will likely lead to improved care for Black women,[23] and frankly any woman against whom we may hold implicit biases. Can we begin to repair some of the damages that have been done to African American women? Can we reverse the epigenetic effects, lengthen the shortened telomeres, put an end to the political, and social marginalization? Can we make childbirth safer for Black women in America? Can we eliminate the health disparities? I have multiple reasons to believe that the answer is: Absolutely yes! It will take financial investments and time. It will take institutional and political will. It will take individual effort, but it can be done.

African Americans have paved the way for people like me to be in America. They have paved the way for outstanding Black people who were immigrants or had immigrant parents like Yvette Francis-McBarnette, Shirley Chisholm, Sidney Poitier, Harry Belafonte, Colin Powell, Barack Obama, Kamala Harris, and so many more. Yet they never received their forty acres and a mule. Even when they thrived, multiple deliberate efforts were made to thwart their progress. If this country is ready to truly address the wrongs of the past, why not start by allowing African American babies the best start possible by fully supporting their mothers during the critical periods of their babies' development and early lives. As an obstetrician, it is hard for me to think of a better way to start repairing the damage of the past than starting at the very beginning of a life. Certainly, much more is needed, but this I believe would be one powerful route.

CHAPTER 2

Black Women and Fertility—How Is the System Failing Them?

Emma White* had been seeing Dr. Frank, her obstetrician-gynecologist (OB/GYN) for the past few years for her routine Pap smear, but this time her request was very different. Emma held a leadership position at a local university. She met Anthony, her husband, about a year and a half before. They discussed their shared desire to have children early in their relationship, and though during their first year of intimacy they did nothing to prevent pregnancy, their attempts moved into high gear during the first few months after their wedding. She had been tracking her periods, since they had sometimes been irregular, using ovulation predictor kits, which she had learned about because of the openness of some of her White girlfriends who had fertility struggles. She and her husband paid particular attention to the timing of intercourse. Detail-oriented and research-minded by nature, she was aware of the possible difficulties she could have in achieving pregnancy as she approached her thirty-seventh birthday.

But Dr. Frank heard none of her concerns. She disregarded Emma's emphatic plea for help. She dismissed all her efforts and research.

"It's because you're stressed out, just relax and enjoy it."

"I know my body." Emma insisted.

"Oh, you're still young, you just got married, just keep trying."

Emma was devastated. The trauma of that visit has remained with her for years, especially because of everything that followed.

---

*Anonymized patient name

The definition of infertility is one year of a couple having unprotected sex without achieving pregnancy.[1] Obstetricians and gynecologists are usually taught to intervene after six months for women thirty-five and over, since fertility is known to decline with age, and thus taking too long to intervene when a woman is older could jeopardize her chances of a successful intervention. Data from the National Survey of Family Growth has shown that there was a downward trend in infertility from 8.5% to 7.4% among married women in America between 1982 and 2002.[2] The gains in fertility were most evident for women between the ages of thirty-five and forty-four. However, when this data was examined by race, the results told a different story. For married White women, the infertility rates improved from 11.6% to 7.1%. Married Black women were not so lucky. Their infertility rate increased from 7.8% to 11.6%. The authors of the survey explained the overall improved fertility rates by the fact that women were potentially starting medical fertility treatment sooner; however, while they noted that a disparity existed for Black women, they did not offer any explanation.

Building on those findings, another group of researchers decided to evaluate any differences in the fertility between Black and White women, including both married and unmarried women in four US cities.[3] Reinforcing the disparity we saw in the other study, Black women were twice as likely to experience infertility when compared to White women. The study also found that Black women who had acknowledged having difficulty paying for the basics had a higher risk of infertility, independent of whether or not they had health insurance. The researchers also found that Black women who had larger ovaries on ultrasound had a higher likelihood of being infertile. This relationship was not observed among White women. The authors noted that large ovaries could be associated with ovarian cyst or other ovarian tissue, and acknowledged that this finding warranted further scientific investigation. While this study did find that Black women were more likely to have fibroids than White women, the presence of fibroids seemed to have a similar impact on the fertility of both Black and White women.

I mentioned in the last chapter some of the evidence which shows that disparities are not related to the intrinsic genetic makeup of Black women. Another study backs this up. In 2021, a group of researchers from well-respected medical institutions in the Northeast specifically evaluated the influence on the ethnicity of Black patients on their diagnosis of infertility.[4] Specifically, they looked at Black American, Black Haitian, Black African, and White American women who sought infertility care at the Boston Medical Center between January 2005 and July 2015. Black or White race was self-identified, and ethnicity was determined by the place of birth and primary language. The researchers excluded ethnically Haitian women who were born in the United States. Black and White American women had their infertility diagnosed at a similar age, but the Black women of the other ethnicities were older. Black women had higher body mass indexes (BMIs), a marker of obesity, with the highest BMIs in Black American women.

Black African women were more likely to be married than any other group, even including White women, and Black American women were the least likely to be married. Black women, even if they were Black American, were more likely to be uninsured or on Medicaid, compared to White American women, 45.5% and 13.6%, respectively.

Fascinatingly, while there were certainly differences between Black Americans and White Americans, according to the authors of the study these two groups had more similar baseline characteristics (e.g., age and whether they had prior children) than Black American women had with Black women of the other two ethnicities. These similarities were also noted in the types of infertility diagnoses they were given. I believe this speaks of the role of the environment, rather than baseline genetic makeup, unless we think that Black American women genetically resemble White American women more than they resemble Black women from the continent of Africa or the country of Haiti. Either way we look at it, I believe it reinforces the point that most of the health disparities experienced by Black women in America are based on the multiple negative consequences they are forced to endure because of only one genetic factor, expression of melanin in their skin tone.

Emma reached out to her friend and family network to find another OB/GYN. Another was recommended. She quickly made an appointment with her new OB/GYN, but had to wait two more months for the date. This time Emma felt she was being heard. "She understood," Emma explained, referring to her new OB/GYN who went as aggressively as she could, to treat Emma, under the limitations of the insurance coverage. "To get things covered under insurance there had to be a specific protocol." Emma underwent three cycles of a fertility drug called Clomid (clomiphene citrate). At that time, approaching 2010, it was the most popular drug for the type of infertility that Emma and many Black women face: infertility from not ovulating regularly enough or at all. Three cycles meant that she got three rounds of treatment which had to be spread over a few months. She did get pregnant with one of the cycles, but she miscarried her baby. She was thirty-eight by the time she was able to start in-vitro fertilization (IVF). For any women facing fertility issues, especially those aged thirty-five or older, two years can feel like a lifetime. Aging is not a friend to egg quality either. Egg quality and the ability to generate a sufficient number of eggs are important aspects of IVF treatment.

Emma loved her reproductive endocrinologist, the specialist who would perform her IVF. He was a Black male doctor in an all-Black-staffed practice. Emma felt cared for and respected—attributes she valued even more highly as she continued to suffer through the trauma she felt after the dismissive comments of her first OB/GYN. She underwent four cycles of IVF. Emma knew that her career growth at the local university was stalled. She knew that, professionally, it was time to move on. However, she stayed, because the insurance her employer provided covered IVF.

IVF is an expensive procedure, but often the only manner many women are able to have children. It is not covered by Medicaid and only variably by private insurance. This barrier adds to the inequities that the already disparate numbers of Black infertile women face in achieving a healthy pregnancy and taking home a baby. It is the recommended method of helping a woman to have a baby if she desires to conceive after undergoing a tubal sterilization procedure.

In the twentieth century, 60,000 people in America were involuntarily sterilized under the flawed ideology that certain people's offspring would not be fit for society.[5] People of color, including African Americans, were disproportionately targeted. In the state of North Carolina, Black women were most likely to be forcibly sterilized from 1937 to 1966.[6] Even as recently as 1997 to 2010, nearly 1,400 sterilizations were performed on women in California prisons. Investigations revealed by the documentary *Belly of The Beast* suggest that the majority of the women were Black and Latina,[7] and that for many the procedure was forced.[8]

Tubal sterilization is disproportionately high among Black women in America, about twice as high as among other ethnic groups, arguably based on factors associated with racism.[9] At least some studies have suggested that Black women are more likely to regret it;[10] specifically, if Black women had tubal sterilization performed over the age of thirty, they were almost three times more likely as White women to want it reversed. While, in recent years, the majority of Black women who have had tubal sterilization have presumably done so by choice, rather than being forced, could societal factors be to blame as well? Hypothetically, if a woman needs to exercise control over her reproduction, but due to economics and misinformation she chooses tubal sterilization, is that really a choice? If she has been led to believe by a healthcare provider with a bias, either implicit or overt, that tubal sterilization is her best option, is that a choice? If she feels pressured to terminate her fertility to avoid negative stereotypes associated with Black women who have larger families, is that a choice?

But what about Black women with other types of fertility issues that have nothing to do with sterilization? Even if Black women have insurance, they are less likely to seek fertility help compared to White women.[11] I think this difference could be related to lack of knowledge, stereotypes, and stigma. I remember when a friend, a Black professional woman, tearfully confided in me about her fertility struggle. She had finally met a partner with whom she wanted to parent. When they couldn't conceive, she discovered that her ovarian function had diminished, even though she was only forty. She was then informed that it is not abnormal for women to lose their ovarian function as early as forty. She was devasted, especially since she had been seeing the same gynecologist for many years. He was a White male who had been the obstetrician for her sister and had been a "good doctor." Yet he never told her that her childbearing abilities diminished with age. He never educated her on the fact that the regular periods that she was seeing on the birth control pill were not an indicator of ovarian function, since her pill was blocking ovulation. Even when he gave her the diagnosis, instead of discussing other options, including donor egg, which had already been available for years, he emphasized her low likelihood of success and the costliness of IVF.

Then there are the issues of stigma and stereotypes. If society leads you to believe that you should not only be fertile but super fertile, if society ties your worth to your ability to produce children as it was in the days of slavery; if your culture dictates that, if you are unable to bear children, there is something innately wrong with you, will you hide it? Will you be afraid to talk about it with your friends or family? Would you be afraid to seek help from a medical system that already has been known to judge you too harshly?

Fortunately, I believe at least this aspect will change. Thanks to the bravery of Michelle Obama who admitted that her daughters were born by IVF: she did so not only in the pages of her book *Becoming* for others to read, but publicly in interviews so that other audiences would know. Thanks to the bravery of Gabrielle Union-Wade who documented her infertility story, including failed IVF attempts and multiple miscarriages, in her book *We're Going to Need More Wine*. I love her words: "I'm so glad I got over myself and my fear of what people would think of me if I did not carry my own child."[12]

Emma has readily admitted that much of her knowledge about the infertility process was acquired through the open sharing of her White girlfriends. The issue just wasn't discussed in the Black community. I can add, based on my experience living in Jamaica, that this embarrassment about sharing fertility struggles is not limited to the Black community in America.

Nevertheless, I don't believe that healthcare should leave it up to famous celebrities to educate Black women about fertility. Increased efforts need to be made by insurers, healthcare institutions, and healthcare clinicians to educate their Black patients about fertility in a culturally appropriate and respectful way. OB/GYNs and other women's health clinicians can easily ask their Black patients about their fertility goals in a non-judgmental and open-ended manner. The question can open the door to further education about age-related changes in fertility and about reproductive technologies, such as egg freezing and IVF.

I remember that, in my years of private practice, fertility was a frequent discussion I had with my patients, particularly if they had reached their thirties. I wanted them to be fully aware that fertility had a timeline, especially for women. I always feel a sense of sadness when I have first-time patient encounters with women who have reached their forties, are interested in fertility, but had never learned that biologically it may already be too late. It seems like I see it more often with my Black patients.

Needless to say, education alone is not enough. Both private and publicly funded federal and state insurance need to expand the infertility benefits for Black women. If equity is truly a goal, the level of funding needs to increase in proportion to the level of the disparities.

I remember when I was more ignorant about the reasons for the disparities Black women experienced, I wondered whether public funding like Medicaid should be used to cover IVF. I don't have that question anymore. If a society basically set someone up to be on Medicaid, like it has done for too many Black women due the lack of investments in education, which jeopardizes the ability to create generational wealth, compounded by disparities in opportunity, to name only a few reasons, why punish them even more by denying them the opportunity to get help to conceive children if they need it? For private insurance it should be even less of a debate.

All of Emma's IVF cycles resulted in her becoming pregnant, but she kept miscarrying, every time by the eighth week. Then it happened: a pregnancy that made it past 8 weeks. Her reproductive endocrinologist proudly told her:

"You have graduated, Emma."

She found an outstanding high-risk-pregnancy doctor. From the first moment, she knew that doctor was different from Dr. Frank. She knew that doctor was special. She began to have frequent ultrasounds. It was a baby girl: her baby girl that she wanted so desperately. But all was not well. Emma's caring and empathetic high-risk-pregnancy doctor solemnly shared the ultrasound findings: her baby's brain was not forming correctly. Her daughter could not survive with the condition. Still, Emma held on to every shred of hope. She still saw her daughter moving actively on the ultrasound.

"Are you sure?" How can we know for sure? Her high-risk doctor patiently and compassionately addressed each of Emma's concerns. Emma never felt dismissed or that the information was "dumbed down." Emma underwent another test, an amniocentesis, to verify the findings; still, her doctor counseled her that it was best to end the pregnancy. She was torn. Her uncertainty remained when she arrived at the hospital for her termination. She was then informed by the nursing staff that the amniocentesis was inconclusive.

"Wait! I don't want to do this. I change my mind." Her doctor was quickly called to Emma's bedside and performed another ultrasound. This time she did not see her little girl move. She did not hear her little girl's heartbeat. Emma's baby girl had died.

Emma White did not give up. She waited an entire year for a Black donor embryo, a less expensive option than a donor egg. Only one came along, and her reproductive endocrinologist informed her that the quality was not good enough. Emma was not alone in her struggle to find a Black donor—another fertility struggle faced by many Black women.[13] She wondered if the decision to stay with her reproductive endocrinologist was too highly influenced by the particularly deep bond she had formed with him, which was in turn likely influenced by her traumatic experience with Dr. Frank. Would the treatment have worked if she had seen another reproductive endocrinologist? However, she was comforted by seeing pictures of the babies of other friends he had successfully treated. She wondered if she should have used a White embryo. She shared with me an article about a Black couple who had adopted a White baby boy and then given birth to twin girls using White-donor embryos.[14] She blamed herself for not being brave enough to face the likely negative stigma she would have attracted at that time—the stigma of being thought of as her child's nanny or being criticized for not choosing a Black partner. Emma also shared with me a recent *Wall Street Journal* article about another Black woman who, when faced with the scarcity of Black sperm-donors when she decided to parent as a single divorced woman, chose sperm from people of color of different ethnicities.[15]

"Why didn't I have the insight that she did?" Emma wondered. She has not yet had children, and closure has not yet come, but she is hopeful that she will have complete healing and peace. Fertility treatment does not always guarantee that a woman will be a mother, but it is effective for many. I have met Black women in both my professional and personal life who have been successful. I have sometimes had the pleasure to meet their beautiful children. Gabrielle Union-Wade has her beautiful Kaavia. Michelle Obama has her two beautiful daughters, Malia and Sasha. I have the hope for a healthy child for the many Black mothers who struggle with infertility. I still have the hope for Emma to parent children, even if she has lost hope herself.

CHAPTER 3

A Deep Dive into Miscarriages and Why They Affect Black Women More

Ariel Banks* was thirty-three years old, and things were finally falling into place. She had completed her master's degree and was working with a great company in New York City that she enjoyed; she had married her husband a few months earlier; and she was doing her best to ensure that she was keeping healthy, because she and her husband were ready to start a family. She was surprised when she began to experience pain in her abdomen. She saw her gynecologist, and the diagnosis was great. She was pregnant. Both she and her husband welcomed the news, and he did his best to support her in her healthy lifestyle. The pain went away, and a few weeks later Ariel had an ultrasound which showed an 8-week pregnancy. All was going well. She felt the usual symptoms of pregnancy, including morning sickness, and was excited that her baby was developing inside her.

A few weeks later, something felt wrong. She stopped feeling her pregnancy symptoms. A few days after that, she again had cramping in her lower abdomen. At first, she thought it was normal but when she started to have bleeding, she knew it was not. She did not confide in her husband at first, because she did not want to alarm him. She called her regular obstetrician, but he was on vacation. She then called a physician friend who advised her to go the ER. She went to the ER of the hospital that her doctor worked with, a prestigious hospital on the Upper East Side. She explained her symptoms to the White triage nurse. She was struck by the nurse's annoyed demeanor and even more so by the statement that followed: "Why didn't you stay home and take Tylenol?" The doctor then saw her, and the repeat ultrasound showed that despite being now 13 weeks pregnant, the baby had not progressed beyond 8 weeks, and a miscarriage was inevitable. She could allow the pregnancy to pass naturally or have a dilation and curettage—a process where the contents of the uterus are emptied after a miscarriage, usually performed using a suction device. She chose the latter, and her doctor's covering obstetrician promptly came in and performed the procedure. She was terribly distraught and cried in the recovering room. She felt like her world was coming to an end and was afraid that she would never have a healthy baby. The nurse returned and asked coldly, "Are you crying because you lost the baby or because you are in pain?" Further pained by the coldness and lack of empathy of the nurse, Ariel replied, "What the hell do you think?" The nurse left her room and never returned.

A few days later, her husband had to go on a business trip. He offered to stay, but she assured him that she was fine. But she underestimated her mental state. She was in her eleven-story apartment all alone. Suddenly, she found herself overlooking her balcony railing. She had no recollection of how she got there. It was totally out of her character because she had a fear of heights and would normally avoid the balcony. She promptly realized her vulnerability and packed her bags and went to stay with her nearby in-laws until her husband returned.

Fortunately, two years later she gave birth to a healthy baby, and two years after that her second baby followed. It has been almost eighteen years since Ariel's miscarriage. As painful as it was to lose her baby, she still vividly remembers the cold treatment that she experienced from the nurse.

In the United States, miscarriage is defined as the loss of a pregnancy before 20 weeks of gestation.[1] Most miscarriages are not preventable, since in at least half of the cases of miscarriage, the fetus has a chromosomal abnormality. The overall risk of miscarriage is about 15% for diagnosed pregnancies, but the risk changes with the age of the mother. Women have the lowest risk of 12% if they are aged twenty to twenty-nine and the highest risk, 65%, if they are forty-five or older. An individual woman's risk is lowest if she has never had a miscarriage, but increases by about 10% every time she has a miscarriage, up to 42% if she has had three or more.[2] Black women have a higher rate of miscarriage compared to White women, especially between 10 and 20 weeks of pregnancy,[3] a difference which remained constant even after the researchers accounted for any potential biases in the data.

Risk factors for miscarriage include environmental factors and exposures, acute and chronic stress, as well as medical conditions such and obesity and diabetes. While obesity and diabetes might be more prevalent in Black women, experts suggest that the higher rates of miscarriage for Black women are likely related to the "cumulative stressors of systemic racism, social determinants of health and unavoidable occupational and/or environmental exposure to potential toxins than a true biologic difference."[4]

Taking their cue, I'd like to examine a little further some of these factors that disproportionately affect Black women. Multiple studies have shown that increased exposure to air pollution is associated with an increased risk of miscarriage.[5] In 2009, researchers in California published a report in which not only did African American women have a higher percentage of miscarriages compared to White women, but they found that African Americans were about three times as likely to miscarry if they lived within the highest traffic areas, compared to the lowest traffic areas.[6] This association did not hold for White women or other races studied including Asian or Hispanic women. The only other factor which was found to affect the risk in this study was being a nonsmoker. Nonsmokers also had a higher risk of miscarriage if they lived within these highest traffic areas compared to the lowest traffic areas. In other words, like African Americans, nonsmokers were more vulnerable to effects of air pollution on their early pregnancies. However, for nonsmokers, the excess risk of miscarriage between the highest and lowest traffic areas was about one-and-a-half times compared to the greater than three times risk for African Americans. Furthermore, according to this study, African Americans were no more likely to live in areas with higher levels of traffic than women of other races. A fascinating finding from this study was that smokers were less likely to miscarry if they lived in high traffic areas. Obviously, this is not to say that smoking is protective of miscarriage in general because research has shown that it raises the risk,[7] but rather that certain at-risk behaviors may be protective in at-risk environments. The authors of the report attempted to explain the finding by citing research that

demonstrated that the lung function of smokers was less affected by
pollution than the lung function of nonsmokers.

While the true cause of the disparity between Black and other
women couldn't be determined by this report, the authors wondered
whether nutrition, as measured by lower average intakes of many vita-
mins, could cause that increased susceptibility to harmful air pollution.
Or, I wonder, could epigenetic effects or acute and chronic stressors be
the mediator? Whatever the cause, knowing this increased propensity
of African American women to miscarry when exposed to certain types
of pollutants, it is further disheartening to know that people of color
in America, specifically, Black, Hispanic, and Asians, are disproportionately exposed to fine particulate air pollution.[8] Again, the disparity
is the greatest for Black people. Like in so many other cases, income
was still not protective, since the disparity between people of color
and White people was 2.4 times the range of exposure across income
levels within the specific racial or ethnic subgroup. The factors that
the researchers hold responsible include what they describe as racist
housing policy. This is not the only way that air pollution can potentially affect the miscarriage rate for Black women.

It is well known that Black women are disproportionately affected by
uterine fibroids when compared to White women. Furthermore, Black
women are more likely to be diagnosed with fibroids at younger ages,[9]
in their reproductive years. These fibroids can further increase their risk
of miscarriage.[10] Air pollution in the form of ozone is linked to uterine
fibroids in Black women. The higher the exposure to ozone, the higher
the risk of fibroids. This association was even stronger for women under
thirty-five and further increased for women under thirty.[11] So not only
are Black women at a higher risk of miscarriage and uterine fibroids
due to certain types of air pollution, they now have to contend with this
potentially cumulative effect.

Then there's the question of stress. Some researchers, aware of
conflicting data, were determined to ascertain whether there was a
link between psychologic stress and an increased risk of miscarriage.
To that end, they carried out a systematic review and meta-analysis
which was published in 2017. They identified eight studies which met all
their criteria. After their evaluation was complete, they concluded that
psychological stress, "including life events and occupational stress,"

both before and during pregnancy, was linked to an increased risk of miscarriage.[12] While they used another study to define the experience of stress as situations which "overwhelm" one's "ability to cope,"[13] they acknowledged that the "experience of stress varies, not only by an individual's internal resources but also by the social and material support which is available to them."[14]

Delving into some of the studies reviewed, I discovered some thought-provoking research. One of the studies cited examined the effect of job stress and adverse pregnancy outcome. In designing the questionnaire that they used to assess the impact of job stress, the researchers specifically emphasized the objective nature of work as opposed to the participants' reaction to the work. They found an increased likelihood of miscarriage in jobs with the characteristics of high demand and low control.[15] Another cited study looked at life events and miscarriage risk among a group of women in an inner-city health district in Manchester, United Kingdom. It found that the people in the miscarriage group had significantly fewer social contacts, as defined by people they knew and spoke with regularly; they were significantly less likely to have a "truly intimate" relationship with their partners; and they had a significantly higher likelihood of experiencing a "severe life event" in the 13 weeks before the miscarriage, a higher likelihood of experiencing a "major social difficulty" during the 13 weeks leading up to the miscarriage, and a higher likelihood of experiencing "severe short-term threat" during any of the 3 weeks leading up to the miscarriage.[16] While the stressful life events were not specifically described, the study was based on a frequently used measure of psychological stress that relies on objective measures of the "contextual threat," rather than the woman's subjective report of the "severity of the stressor." While despite these studies there is still some debate about whether psychological stress can impact miscarriage risk, I think that these findings leave little room for debate for Black women.

Let's look at job stressors. Black women are more likely to work in low-paying service jobs.[17] For example, in healthcare, they are more likely to work in some of the "most dangerous and lowest wage jobs."[18] These include jobs such as nurses' aides and licensed practical nurses— jobs with little autonomy, high physical demand, and substantial occupational risk, as the Covid-19 pandemic has shown. That would certainly fit in the category of high demand, low control, which have been shown to increase miscarriage risk. It's hardly likely that this risk is only relegated to Black women in low-income jobs; I am confident that high-income professional Black women are not exempt. Black workers constantly face increased scrutiny on the job, compared to their White counterparts; even when they outperform their White counterparts, they still suffer from discrimination.[19] How about "severe life events?" Black women are more likely to experience physical and sexual violence and psychological abuse.[20] Black people also disproportionately experience homelessness.[21] I am sure lack of a permanent dwelling would fit another category of psychosocial stressors described in the study about life events and miscarriage. Furthermore, for reasons I will discuss later in the book, I suspect Black women will be less likely to report having a "truly intimate" relationship with the father of their babies.

We know that Black women are more likely to experience miscarriages. We know of specific factors that exacerbate the risk. What can be done right now to help? Let's start with air pollution. Governments, NGOs, and corporate entities need to continue to enhance their investment in protecting the environment, a problem that extends far beyond Black women and has implications for our health now and the health of all our children, no matter their race.

That's not all we can do.

Education programs should be targeted to Black women and Black communities not only to improve these communities' understanding of the potential risk of environmental exposures but to arm them with information about steps that they can take to mitigate the risk of exposure: for example, as suggested by Laumbach et al. staying indoors and keeping children indoors on days where the levels of air pollution are higher.[22] Where possible, people should avoid higher-traffic areas when planning their vehicle travel, walking, or exercise routes. Recognizing that economics may limit the mitigation efforts of many Black communities, additional support can be provided through the supply of portable air filtration systems which can reduce indoor pollution levels whether the origins of the pollutants are indoor or outdoor.

We can enhance the support for Black women who are interested in bearing children. Not just for those who have difficulty conceiving but for those who do not. We should expand our outreach to Black women so that they have a greater understanding of the potential benefits of pre-conception counseling. If they have health conditions that are known to impact their pregnancy risk, for example diabetes and hypertension, treatment options can be optimized prior to any attempt to achieve pregnancy. Healthcare workers should ensure that, if needed, Black women receive the appropriate diagnosis and treatment for any fibroids that could affect their miscarriage risk. They should ensure that any medical conditions are appropriately treated, including any unmet mental health needs. The healthcare workforce needs to be sufficiently educated to allow them to meet the needs of their Black patients. Furthermore, Black women need to be educated on the available options to seek the necessary health-insurance coverage even prior to pregnancy; and affordable coverage needs to be made available in the pre-conception period. For too many, insurance coverage that begins after a woman is already pregnant is too late.

Pro-life movements appear to target their interventions exclusively on preventing women from having abortions; how about investing resources in reducing women's risk of miscarriage?

However, all of that might still not be enough if issues of violence against Black women, homelessness, and job discrimination, in terms of both wages and treatment, are not addressed. The stressors that many Black women face far exceed even the most robust coping abilities. Let's stop expecting Black women to fix themselves without giving them the tools.

Early in my career I was on call. It was close to midnight, when a patient came into the emergency room. She was bleeding excessively—so much so that the situation was nearly life-threatening. I needed to immediately empty her uterus of any remains of the already lost pregnancy to avoid further risk to her life. That meant performing a suction dilation and curettage. I had met her previously at her place of business, but learned more about her that evening. Abby Klein* was a talented small-business owner, as such, keeping herself insured was difficult, and the Affordable Care Act was not yet in place. She desperately wanted to have a baby; so much so that she continued to try, when many others would have given up. This was her sixth loss. I would never have known the burden she was carrying, were it not for my role as her physician that night. She always seemed to have it so together. I wanted her to succeed in having a baby, could I direct her to others who could help? I recognized it was beyond my expertise.

Perhaps naively, I discussed all the textbook options. She could see a specialist who deals with recurrent miscarriages, they could help. She seemed open to my suggestion, but I never knew if she was able to procure the resources to see one. Even if she were, the treatment costs could remain prohibitive.

Many years later I checked on her through someone we both knew. Abby shared her story, including my role in her care that night.

She had become a stepmother, but was never able to give birth to any biological children.

"She tried, but it never worked out."

As I write this, I wonder if we are really doing enough for any woman who has a miscarriage. There hardly seems to be sufficient mental health support in place. Is that 2-week visit after the miscarriage enough? I don't wonder whether we are doing enough for Black women. I know we are not. Inequities that have exacerbated environmental exposures and acute and chronic stressors are still in place. For some, the very painful loss is further amplified by insensitive actions or words of healthcare providers bearing explicit or implicit biases against them. I am no longer so naive to think we in healthcare can help all women who miscarry to have a successful pregnancy, but I hope it is as clear to you as it is to me that we can easily do more.

CHAPTER 4

Navigating the Healthcare System—The Added Burden

I have never really reflected on how I chose my OB/GYNs over the years, but as I wrote this book, memories flooded back. My first encounter with a gynecologic exam was at a student health clinic; I recall it being part of our mandatory requirements for a physical. Actually, I'm not sure if the doctor was specifically a gynecologist or one of the allied primary-care specialties. But I do remember this: he was an elderly White man. He was not unkind, he almost had a fatherly manner, as awkward or even creepy as that word might sound in this context. The encounter was awkward and maybe a little bit creepy. I remember him asking "do you have a boyfriend?" The answer was no. Without much further explanation, he proceeded to do a Pap smear. I remember feeling almost violated, although I know that was not his intent. There was no question about whether I had ever been sexually active: I wasn't. There was no discussion about why the Pap test was needed. There was nothing. I never shared this experience with anyone until after I started writing it down. Even though I knew Pap smears were recommended yearly at that time for women of my age, whether or not one was sexually active, I don't recall visiting another gynecologist until residency. I was traumatized, but I didn't even realize it. In residency, choosing a gynecologist was a little awkward for various reasons. It is uncomfortable to visit someone you work with personally for such an intimate exam, but at the same time it is preferential to go to someone you respect clinically. The obvious choice was from among the doctors I worked with. Maybe instinctively I chose a woman. I'm not sure if my choice was guided by that first experience. I chose a Black female OB/GYN, thankfully not hard to find in Washington, DC, where I did my training. Why a Black woman? I didn't really know. At the time, I didn't think that the race of my doctor would matter to me. The person I chose was a good instructor, but she did not have a particularly charismatic or effervescent personality. But I felt safe with her, and I trusted her medical judgment.

My choice for an obstetrician was relatively easy. This time, I chose a man despite generally feeling more comfortable with female OB/GYNs. He was one of my partners from my first job after residency. He had become a dear friend who warmly welcomed me into his family when I worked with him. I became well acquainted with his wife and two daughters who were young children at the time. He too shared my Caribbean background. My husband had met him a few times on our visits to Florida and also held him in high regard. Another friend whom I had referred to him prior to my pregnancy glowed about his care. I trusted his care implicitly.

At no time during those early years did I have any understanding about implicit bias. I already knew racism still existed in the United States, but I had expected doctors and nurses to be unbiased and caring, at least to their patients, even if they were not always that way to me.

But maybe on an unconscious level I had learned whom to trust. There were still many White male physician instructors and colleagues whose clinical judgment I also trusted and respected. Perhaps that first experience had compromised my comfort with seeking one for OB/GYN care despite my comfort in other areas of medicine.

Choosing whom to go to for OB/GYN care is often a predicament for women—a predicament often worse for Black women in America due to the racism and biases they often face. I have read and heard countless stories of Black women across socioeconomic lines who have been disparaged, berated, and had their concerns minimized by their doctors or other healthcare providers. A physician or a practice or healthcare facility could be highly recommended by a White friend, but for a Black woman the experience could be dehumanizing, even deadly. A gynecologic exam is intimate and deeply personal. Obstetric care has huge implications. Obstetricians spearhead the care in arguably one of the most important seasons of a woman's life, nurturing a developing baby.

The trauma from a negative care experience can last for years; it can last a lifetime. It still haunts Emma White. It still brings her pain—pain that has been eased by subsequent positive experiences, but the scar remains.

In making the choice of OB/GYN, some people have gender preferences. Black women may desire to have someone of their own race. About 5% of physicians in the United States are Black—split almost evenly between men and women.[1] According to US census data, 13.4% of the US population is Black.[2] Interestingly, a significantly larger percentage of Black physicians, 11.1%,[3] enter the field of OB/GYN, but that still leaves less than half a percent of Black OB/GYNs to take care of Black women who make up about 7% of the US population. Why might a Black patient prefer a Black physician? I suspect it is related to some of my reasons. As human beings, we naturally tend to be attracted to people who are like us. For some of us, it is race, ethnicity, or nationality, or a combination of all three. But I realize that for African Americans, or other Black people who have lived in America for a while, there are other reasons. Could they trust them? I am confident that many of my non-Black physician colleagues can deliver unbiased care and am cognizant that some of my Black physician colleagues do not; but in making a choice you want the odds to be stacked in your favor, and I suspect that is the reason for the choice of many Black women.

Unfortunately, many Black women in America do not have a choice. Medicaid covers 65% of births to Black mothers,[4] and it is more widely accepted, in 90% of community health centers and clinics, compared to 77% of private practices.[5] Furthermore, 46% of people on Medicaid get their care at community clinics compared to 24% who get their care at private practices.

That's only part of the problem. In 2017, more than half of US counties were in need of an OB/GYN[6]—a problem that is only projected to worsen due to an undersupply of more than 5,000 full-time OB/GYNs by 2030.[7] Conversely, the supply of certified nurse midwives is expected to exceed the demand. Why might that be a problem when it is recognized that midwives are commonly underutilized in the US healthcare system? For reasons I have and will continue to discuss, Black women may face more risk factors entering pregnancy or develop more complications during pregnancy, while midwives are generally trained to care for low-risk pregnancies. Neither patients nor clinicians are well served if the risk level of the patient is incompatible with the skill set of the clinicians.

For community health centers and clinics, the problem appears to be amplified. In my many years of experience serving in these settings, I have observed many of the patients having high risk factors; yet I believe that the time allotted to see them is often too limited. To compound this, due to physician shortages, midwives and other advanced-practice practitioners (APPs) are sometimes compelled to see higher acuity patients, while having limited opportunities to consult with physicians who are often faced with similar or greater time constraints.

This disparity extends to hospital systems. In 2018, Dr. Elizabeth A. Howell, a graduate of Harvard Medical School and current chair of the Department of Obstetrics and Gynecology at University of Pennsylvania Perelman School of Medicine,[8] published a manuscript highlighting the effect that the quality of the delivery hospital has on morbidity and mortality for Black women.[9] Dr. Howell is a nationally recognized expert on quality of care and health disparities for both maternal and infant health.

She observed some remarkable findings. Seventy-five percent of Black women delivered in 25% of hospitals, while only 18% of White women delivered in those same hospitals. The reason that is particularly problematic is that the likelihood of having complications is higher in these hospitals, whether the woman is Black or White, even after adjusting for risk factors. When Dr. Howell and her team applied a model to estimate the cost of that excess risk to Black pregnant women in New York City, they estimated that almost 1,000 fewer women would have avoided a major complication based on the 2011–2013 data analyzed. The net outcome: patients who sometimes need the highest level of care get the least.

Even if a Black woman doesn't necessarily need the highest level of care, even if she is well-educated and has resources, even if she is healthy, her pregnancy planned, and her insurance allows her to choose the most well-respected OB/GYNs in the area, she may still worry about navigating her prenatal care and her delivery. In fact, a research study published in 2000 confirmed why she might worry. Examining data from pregnancy-related deaths in the entire United States and Puerto

Rico from 1979 to 1986, including Black and White Hispanic women, Saftlas et al. found the largest Black–White racial disparity in maternal deaths among Black women who had the lowest risk.[10] Black women who gave birth to normal-birthweight babies, had three or fewer children, and did not have any socioeconomic disadvantages were significantly more likely to die than their White counterparts. Conversely, at least at that time, Black and White women who gave birth to low birthweight babies and had four or more children were equally likely to die.

Kira Johnson was an accomplished businesswoman in education and hospitality.[11] She spoke five languages and had a pilot's license.[12] She died twelve hours after an elective cesarean section at Cedars-Sinai Hospital, ten hours after her doctor was notified of a problem.[13]

I feel sad when young professional Black women who want to have children confide in me that they are worried or scared. I feel sad that any Black woman has to be worried or scared because they know that the system they have to navigate could be, in some ways, a minefield.

There are solutions. A few that I will suggest are based on my own experience. Health centers, clinics, and hospitals where the majority of Black women seek care and deliver need more resources. They need resources to attract skilled obstetricians. They need resources so that those skilled doctors have adequate time for the prenatal visits. These resources can be obtained if Medicaid and other insurers increase the compensation rate for the visits or organizations provide grants to subsidize the clinic operations or both if the aim is really to eliminate the disparities as is often claimed. If strong bonds are formed between the patient and their obstetric clinician, continuity should be a priority. The care centers should have avenues for their Black patients to safely disclose if they do not feel comfortable with the care they are receiving and provide options.

Similarly, the hospitals need the resources as well so that they can attract talented OB/GYNs. OB/GYNs who are open to midwifery care and doula support. OB/GYNs should be allowed easy access to the required specialist to partner with in the delivery of care for any pregnant or postpartum patient who may have additional risks. Almost three-quarters of OB/GYNs who accept Medicaid report challenges in finding a specialist for their Medicaid patients, compared to their privately insured patients.[14] The hospitals need resources so that they have the equipment to diagnose life-threatening pregnancy-related conditions, as well as develop the expertise and acquire the facilities and the equipment to treat them.

I remember the one time a patient's heart stopped on my operating table. I was doing a routine cesarean section. She was a Black pregnant woman. I don't remember any cause or warning sign. What I do remember is the team of anesthesiologists working at the time. They knew what to do and intervened quickly. They restored her normal heartbeat, and I was able to complete the surgery without difficulty. The patient recovered and was able to have the proper evaluation she needed to rectify the problem.

I remember another time when a young Latina woman came into the hospital with high blood pressure late in her pregnancy. It was on my shift. Before her diagnosis of preeclampsia could be confirmed, she had an eclamptic seizure. Even though I knew the recommended seizure medication, magnesium sulfate, I remember the internal medicine team coming immediately to the patient's bedside to assist me and help to ensure her seizures were well controlled. The patient went on to have a vaginal delivery, but she suffered from postpartum hemorrhage (life-threatening bleeding after delivery). Despite employing every method at my disposal, I could not stop the bleeding on my own. I knew that taking the patient to the operating theater could be very dangerous: she could lose her uterus; she could have uncontrollable bleeding. But I had a choice. I had access to the interventional radiologist whom I had alerted earlier when my concerns were growing and my interventions were failing. He came in and performed a procedure called uterine artery embolization. Blocking agents were introduced into the patient's blood vessels and guided to the uterine vessels where the bleeding needed to be controlled. The procedure worked. It saved my patient's life, and it saved her uterus. Outstanding resources are available at many US hospitals. Outstanding doctors are available at many US practices. But these same practices and well-resourced hospitals are sometimes places of turmoil for Black women—Black women who know that all the advantages may exist in those settings, that their insurance allows them ready access, but wonder if they will be ignored or mistreated. Will being ignored lead them to have major complications? Will being ignored cost them their lives?

How do Black women know which doctors or other healthcare professionals will see her as a person first? Word of mouth from trusted Black friends or colleagues may help. What if you have no one to ask?

Kimberly Seals Allers, an award-winning journalist, bestselling author, speaker, and advocate, has sought to provide a way.[15] Based on her own traumatic experience of feeling "disrespected," "ignored," and "violated" as an unwed Black mother having her first child in a New York City hospital, she created the Irth app. It didn't matter that the student insurance she was on was from Columbia University or that she had just completed her master's degree. Frankly, it should not have mattered. She should have been treated with respect, regardless; but it just provides another example of how Black women cannot educate themselves out of the mistreatment. The app allows Black and brown "birthing people" to view and provide ratings and reviews of maternity and pediatric doctors and delivery hospitals. Generous donors, such as the Tara Foundation, the California Health Foundation, and the Grove foundation, have helped Ms. Seals Allers do her important work.

Health is Her Hue is also trying to close the gap. Together with her co-founder Eddwina Bright, Ashlee Wisdom, the CEO, is using her BA in psychology and her master's in public health to make a difference.[16] She recognized a need, based on her experiences growing up in the Bronx, New York, as well as her academic experiences at New York University and professional experiences working in New York City.[17] The goal of Ashlee Wisdom's digital platform is to connect "Black women to the healthcare providers, services and resources that are committed to their health and well-being."[18]

However, these women cannot do their work alone. They need continued investment and resources to improve their innovations and get closer to their goals. As do the community clinics or federally qualified health centers (FQHCs) and the hospitals that serve predominantly Black women. The truth is that none of this work should have been needed; racism should not be the biggest risk factor for Black women as they navigate the health system. But Black pregnant and postpartum women cannot afford to wait for America to act the way it should. Kira Johnson and too many others were not given the luxury of time.

CHAPTER 5

Preterm Birth Story—How the Disparity Perpetuates

I had no choice but to deliver her baby. The fetus was on the edge of viability, about 24 weeks, I knew that chance of survival was low, but with the finding from the antenatal testing by the high-risk obstetrician, if the baby remained inside her body the chance of survival would likely be zero. Her family gathered around her. They were prayerful and hopeful but from my physician's perspective I knew that hope would not be enough. My experience with faith taught me prayers are not always answered in the way we want them to be. The patient in question was an older Black mother who was having her first child. She had high blood pressure, but that did not explain why her baby was growing so poorly inside her and why this only partially developed baby had to be separated from her body so early. I made sure the patient had a chance to see and kiss her baby before he was taken to the neonatal intensive care unit (NICU). I did not know if she ever would be able to see him alive again. She did not.

Preterm birth can be spontaneous or induced. A woman may go into labor well before her due date often without any apparent cause. In other cases, she or her baby may have a medical condition or complication that requires that we, as obstetricians, deliver her baby early. Sometimes even before the full term of 37 weeks, the developing baby is mature enough to avoid any serious consequences of being born prematurely but often it is not. Early preterm births are defined by the Centers for Disease Control and Prevention (CDC) as births that occur at less than 34 weeks of pregnancy and late preterm births occur from 34 to 36 weeks.[1]

In 2020, according to the National Center for Health Statistics (NCHS) data brief, the overall rate of preterm births in the United States was 8.42% if a mother was only carrying a single baby (singleton pregnancy). For non-Hispanic (NH) Black women, the rate was 12.18%, a slight but not statistically significant increase from the 2019 rate of 12.12%. For NH White women the rate declined significantly from 7.44 in 2019 to 7.36 in 2020.[2] These rates go up if multiple gestation pregnancies (a mother carrying two or more babies) are included. This overall rate was 10.1% in 2020, a slight decrease, but again not for Black people who saw a rate of 14.4%.[3] Among other health indicators for maternal and child health, the March of Dimes tracks preterm birth rates. The March of Dimes was established under the leadership of President Franklin D. Roosevelt in his efforts to combat polio, a disease that affected him personally.[4] The organization's original name was the National Foundation for Infant Paralysis. It successfully funded Dr. Jonas Salk in the development of the polio vaccine.[5] Polio has been largely eradicated with successful vaccination programs.[6] After that success, the March of Dimes's mission changed to address other challenges in infant health. More recently, it has broadened its focus to the protection of the health of mothers and babies with an emphasis on prematurity.[7] In addition, its President and CEO, Stacey Stewart, has been a vocal advocate for health equity and reducing the maternal mortality and morbidity crisis for Black mothers and other marginalized groups. Among the preterm birth rate metrics tracked are disparities in rates. According to their data the disparities have worsened.[8] Some states fail Black mothers more than others. In Alabama, the preterm birth rate, based on 2017 to 2019 averages, was 16.1% for Black women, compared to 10.8% for White women. For Louisiana, it was even worse, at 16.6%, with the same rate of 10.8% for White women. Mississippi had the worst rates in the entire country: 12.1% for White women and 17.1% for Black women.

Complications of prematurity are one of the key reasons why babies die,[9] and can lead to multiple health problems even if the infants do live.[10] I followed with fascination the story of Curtis Means, a Black child who, born at 21 weeks and 1 day, is the most premature baby to survive.[11] He was a twin, but his sister died one day after she was born. Many would call Curtis's survival a medical miracle. The medical team rallied around him; he received "round-the-clock" care, and after 275 days was discharged from the University of Alabama at Birmingham Regional Intensive Care Unit and was able to go home to his family. But not without cost. As a parent, I am confident that to Curtis's parents having him alive outweighs any healthcare demands, but due to his prematurity there are demands nonetheless. According to a news story on Yahoo!Life, "[Curtis] still has health challenges and delays—including taking medication for hypertension, being on oxygen, using a gastrostomy, or G-, tube for feeding and requiring on-demand feeds every three hours to build up his calorie intake as an underweight child."[12]

Why is the problem of preterm births so much worse for Black women in America than for White women? A few years ago, Dr. Tracy Manuck, a professor at the University of North Carolina–Chapel Hill, published an article attempting to answer that question.[13] Among the possible explanations she included was socioeconomic factors. While she identified studies confirming that being economically disadvantaged can increase the risk for preterm birth (and low birthweight) for both Black and White mothers, she also found that the impact of being economically disadvantaged was much greater on the preterm birth rates among NH White women than among NH Black women. Specifically, NH White mothers were 48% more likely to experience preterm birth if they lived in the most disadvantaged neighborhoods compared to the least disadvantaged neighborhoods. For low birthweight (LBW) the difference was 61%. For NH Black women, the difference was only 15% for preterm birth and 17% for LBW.[14]

Dr. Manuck then discussed education as a marker of socioeconomic status and cited a study that compared the preterm delivery and low birthweight in children of Black and White college graduates. At the time the study was published, in 1992, it was thought that Black and White college graduates would have similar environmental risk factors. Even after controlling for any variables that they could identify between the graduates, Black female college graduates had a higher risk of delivering preterm (1.28) or having a low-birthweight baby (1.75).[15] Furthermore, Dr. Manuck added that disparities persist even with similar access to healthcare as in military personnel.

Other risks factors, such as smoking, illicit drug use, and certain elements of psychosocial stress, offered little to explain the difference, especially since these specific factors were more common in White women.[16]

While Dr. Manuck noted that genetics can influence preterm birth rates, her research did not reveal any conclusive genetic differences between races that can explained the disparities. She opined that "epigenetics may provide the key to understanding some of the heritability of preterm birth."[17] As I mentioned in chapter 1, the adverse effects of racism can lead to epigenetic changes, which can be passed on to subsequent generations and cause negative effects on their health, effects that can start as early as when they are developing in their mother's uterus.

Multiple researchers have examined the differences in preterm birth rates for US-born NH Black women compared with foreign-born NH Black women. Time and time again, the research has found that the preterm birth rate is lower for foreign-born Black women compared to those born in the United States. A group of researchers decided to dig deeper into the differences by specifically looking at the countries and regions where foreign Black women were born. They continued to find the disparities, with US-born Black women having a 30% higher rate of preterm birth than foreign-born Black women, a difference that remained even after the researchers controlled for any variables such as socioeconomic status, medical risk, or health behaviors.[18] When they further evaluated the preterm birth rate of women born in the Caribbean versus those born in Sub-Saharan Africa (SSA), they noticed the latter had lower preterm birth rates. They also noted that a higher proportion of the women from SSA had emigrated within five years before the data was collected—compared to Caribbean women, three quarters of whom had been in the United States more than ten years— and suggested that the shorter time in the United States meant not only that the women from SSA may be more attached to their traditional values, but they would have "less cumulative exposure to discrimination."[19] Building upon the work of some of this earlier research, we have continued to gain understanding of how racism affects multiple aspects of the lives of Black people, and preterm birth is a part of that list.

In another article, a senior writer at the Population Reference Bureau (PBR), Paola Scommegna, quoted Dr. Catherine Cubbin describing some of the mechanisms of how the stress of racism affects the developing baby.[20] Dr. Cubbin has spent much of her career evaluating racial and ethnic disparities in health.

Ms. Scommegna also highlighted a study that I found particularly innovative. The researchers, Nguyen et al. collected a random 1% sample of public tweets from June 2015 to December 2017.[21] They were able to scientifically categorize racial and ethnic tweets and distinguish whether they were positive or negative, and geographically link the tweets to the US state from which they were posted. The results were compelling. Of the just-under-24-million race- or ethnicity-related tweets, more than 15 million were in reference to Black people and fewer than two million to any of the other groups studied, which included White people, Hispanic people, Asian people, and Middle Eastern people. Mothers who lived in states with the highest level of racial or ethnic tweets had an 8% higher rate of preterm birth and low-birthweight babies. States with more negative tweets targeting Black people correlated with a higher incidence low birthweight and preterm birth in Black mothers. No such correlation existed for White mothers, but one particularly thought-provoking finding showed that a greater number of negative tweets about "racial or ethnic minority groups" were associated with higher rates of preterm birth and low birthweight among NH White women. The negativity was affecting the pregnancy of White women, even though they did not belong to any of the groups that were attacked.

There are initiatives in place trying to combat preterm birth rates. In the same March of Dimes report that I referenced earlier, perhaps the only state that I thought really stood out in terms of the overall diversity and the effectiveness in narrowing the disparity gap in preterm birth rates between Black and White women was Colorado. According to the 2020 Census, 4.6% of people in Colorado were African American or Black.[22] The overall preterm birth rate was 9.1%, with 8.7% for White women and 11.4% for Black women. Of six key indicators and policy actions that March of Dimes monitors to improve the health of moms and babies in the United States, Colorado had implemented four: Medicaid expansion, midwifery policy, maternal mortality review committees (MMRCs), and perinatal quality collaborative. Vermont, the state with the lowest preterm birth rate of 7.6%, at least for White women, since the Black population is small, had also implemented these four. Other states, such as California, have implemented, or plan to implement, all six (the other two being Medicaid extension and doula policy or legislation). While the preterm birth rate for White women is 7.7% in California, the disparity-narrowing benefits for Black women have yet to be seen, with the rate still at 12.2% and a 44% disparity compared to other women. The problem is that, although these initiatives are important and I am confident they will help to improve preterm birth rates overall, they are not enough to eliminate the disparities because they do not cure racism.

I would be disingenuous if I said that I expect racism to be eliminated, but I do think that continuing to own up to, and acknowledge, its effects on Black pregnant women and their families can be helpful. It doesn't help any Black person, and even less so Black pregnant women, to be blamed for the outcomes of racism or being told that their perceptions of the racism they continue to experience are incorrect. Colorado appears to be acknowledging the impact of racism. The recommendations issued by Colorado Department of Public Health and Environment start by recognizing the chronic stress African American women endure due to lifelong exposure to racial discrimination.[23] The recommendations also highlight the protective advantage that immigrant African women have, but note that it is lost after only one generation, when their daughters have children.

Black pregnant women also need to be armed with additional tools to cope. As the March of Dimes suggests, all barriers to access care need to be eliminated. Housing and childcare support for Black pregnant women should be fortified. Other strategies that have proven to be effective in reducing preterm birth should be implemented or enhanced.

Researchers at Emory and Yale universities conducted a randomized control trial to evaluate group prenatal care due to promising non-randomized studies showing its benefits in reducing preterm birth and low birthweight.[24] Randomization is considered the gold standard for evaluating any particular intervention because it is designed to reduce research bias. The participants ranged in age from fourteen to twenty-five years old. Eighty percent of the participants were African American. Thirty-eight percent of the participants had completed high school, 36% were still in high school, 26% had dropped out, and 31% were employed. The participants in the group prenatal care had a preterm birth rate of 9.8% versus 13.8% in the individual care group. When the study specifically looked at the rates for African American women, the researchers discovered a 10% preterm birth rate for those in group care versus 15.8% for those who were not in group care. They were able to analyze the cost for the Yale cohort and found no difference in cost between the groups.

Group prenatal care is not necessarily easy to implement and requires institutional buy-in. Public funding and support would be beneficial. I refuse, however, to believe that it cannot be effectively used to decrease preterm birth rates for Black women. Implementation of group prenatal care requires the consideration of group dynamics and patients need to feel safe in any group in which they participate. As such, the organizers should consider the age and socioeconomic demographics of the group members. Group prenatal visits might be better suited for locations which care for predominantly Black women of similar socioeconomic status.

In 2021, a literature review specifically sought to identify interventions to reduce preterm birth and stillbirth in low- and middle-income countries. In multiple studies, micronutrient supplementation was effective in reducing the rate of preterm birth.[25] While the United States is not a low- or middle-income country, it is certainly no secret that the typical American diet and the diet being eaten by many African Americans lacks in nutritional content. Additional investigation should be done to determine whether micronutrient supplementation would be safe and effective for reproductive-age Black women who are at risk for dietary deficiencies in pregnancy.

We should not rely on supplements alone. Measures can be initiated immediately to improve the diet of Black pregnant women. A meta-analysis published in 2019 using pooled data from six studies concluded that a healthy dietary pattern—described as high intake of vegetables, fruits, whole grains, low-fat dairy, and lean protein foods—reduced the risk of preterm birth.[26] Women in the "top tertile of healthy dietary patterns" had a 21% risk reduction compared to women in the lowest tertile. Adding to these findings, a randomized control study evaluating a cholesterol-lowering diet among nonsmoking White pregnant women in Norway found a statistically significant decrease in preterm birth among the women on the diet versus women who were consuming their usual diet.[27] The study deliberately focused on low-risk pregnant women but excluded women who were vegetarian or on a Mediterranean-type diet. Interestingly, the intervention which consisted of dietary advice from a dietician at entry into the study, 24, 30, and 36 weeks, was started at 17–20 weeks. Participants were recruited after they had a normal 17–20 week ultrasound exam. As it is in the United States, an ultrasound at about that gestational age is the standard of care in Norway. The dietary recommendations included fatty fish, vegetable oils with an emphasis on olive and rapeseed oil, nut butters, avocadoes to replace meat, butter, cream, and fatty dairy product. The participants were advised to have at least six fresh fruits and vegetables daily. They were allowed to have meat for a main meal twice a week and on the other main dishes they were to use "legumes, vegetable main dishes, fatty fish or poultry with the fat trimmed off." They were even given cooking lessons on foods that they may have been less familiar with. The difference was remarkable. Eleven of the 149 women in the control group had a preterm delivery compared to one of the 141 women in the intervention group.

I found this intervention particularly exciting because, even if we do not get to intervene in the care of a Black pregnant woman until after the first trimester, a potentially very large impact can still be made in reducing her likelihood of a preterm delivery by just helping her to improve her diet.

In developed countries, namely Australia, Canada, Ireland, and the United Kingdom, midwifery-led models of care have been shown to reduce the rates of preterm birth.[28] As I mentioned earlier in this chapter, access to midwifery care has been acknowledged by the March of Dimes as an important step to improving maternal health. I do think this has potential for Black women as long as they are cared for by midwives who do not hold negative biases against them, either implicit or explicit. Facilitating the training of midwives who are already motivated to serve Black communities could be one way to ensure that this workforce is available. Midwifery care by Black and/or other culturally sensitive midwives has other potential benefits for Black mothers which I will discuss later in this book.

There is something else we might be able to do to help reduce the rates of preterm birth in Black women: educate Black men. In a research article published in 2021, Dr. Paris Ekeke and colleagues attempted to further explain the disparities in preterm birth rate between US-born and foreign-born Black women, since differences in maternal education did little to explain the disparities. They sought to investigate the impact of the father's education on the preterm birthrate of foreign-born Black women, and specifically looked at the educational attainment of the fathers whose paternity was acknowledged. In the sample which included data from the 2013 US natality files from the National Center for Health Statistics, the preterm birth rate for US-born Black women was 13.3%, compared to 10.8% for foreign-born Black women. For both the US-born and foreign-born Black women the rate of preterm birth decreased if the fathers had higher levels of education, from less than high school to high school diploma/GED, to some college or an associate degree, to a bachelor's degree, to a master's degree, or higher. After adjusting for other factors, including maternal education, the father's education accounted for almost 15% of the difference in preterm birth rate between the groups compared to under 4% for maternal education. We can't cure racism, but improving the educational attainment in the Black community, not only of the women but also the Black men who are most likely to be the fathers, is another intervention that can help to give Black babies a better start in life.

It was in my first job out of residency: I was part of a group that provided obstetric and gynecologic hospital services for Broward General Hospital. I was still in my first year there when one of my lifelong friends became pregnant with her first child. I had had the privilege of serving as a bridesmaid at her wedding a few years earlier. One night I got an urgent call. Her water had broken. Her pregnancy was only at 31 weeks. We were not confident of the likelihood that her daughter would survive if she was born that early in a Jamaican healthcare facility, given the neonatal intensive care facilities available at that time (more than twenty years ago). I was certain that Broward General Hospital had the facilities. Fortunately, the hospital accepted the transfer of care. My friend was brought to Broward General by air ambulance, and I was able to care for her: having a close friend under one's care is a difficult situation to be in, but I knew I was in a position to give her baby girl the best chance she could get.

While the flight between Fort Lauderdale and Kingston is relatively short, under two hours, air ambulance can cost several thousand US dollars, a cost that is a great sacrifice for most and prohibitive for many.

My friend and her husband were willing to do anything they could possibly do to save their daughter, no matter the sacrifice. I know of other mothers who have braved commercial flights with potentially life-threatening pregnancy conditions to give their developing babies the best possible care.

We admitted my friend and hoped that the baby would stay in the womb a few weeks longer. Only a few days later she went into labor. Since her daughter was breech, I performed a cesarean section. The baby girl weighed three pounds and had to remain in the NICU for 6 weeks. I was bestowed the additional honor of being named her godmother. My goddaughter is a beautiful, healthy, talented girl. I will be forever grateful for the care and facilities at Broward General Hospital, which helped to ensure that she got the very best start despite being born so early. I am grateful that the United States has many such facilities to save preterm babies, but I know that mothers and babies alike would be better off if we could reduce the number of instances when those advanced facilities are needed. We can do so by bringing down the rates of preterm birth in the United States, an outcome we will not be able to achieve unless we give Black pregnant women the helping hand they need.

CHAPTER 6

Multiple Gestation—How Many Black Babies Will Survive?

I used to dream of having twins. When I was growing up, I wanted to have four children, like my maternal grandmother, two boys and two girls just as she had. I felt that it was important that each child have a companion close to their age, and I figured twins were a great way to ensure that. My maternal grandmother gave birth to my mother and her identical twin sister in Jamaica when she was forty-one years old. She then lived for another fifty-eight years. With that as my example I would never have imagined the risks that were associated with the delivery of even one baby, much less multiples.

Even after I decided to pursue obstetrics and learned more about the risk of childbirth, I didn't completely let go of my childhood desire, but was nonetheless grateful, and maybe a little relieved, that my two babies came one at a time. Given my late start to childbearing, and knowing that I had to balance the responsibility of having to work to help to provide the life I wanted for my children with the need and desire to spend time with them, I gave up on my wish to expand my family any further. But for someone who has been struggling with infertility, twins must have felt like a Godsend. It took my grandmother about fifteen years to finally get pregnant with a baby; she then had each of my uncles, and afterward, her precious girls, my mother and her twin sister. I never thought to ask her how it felt when her two girls were born or even if she knew that she was carrying more than one baby.

Dr. Oneeka Williams knew she was carrying twins. They were the culmination of a long struggle with infertility and four cycles of IVF, and she did everything she could to care for her precious cargo. As a physician, she had more than a passing knowledge of the risks that could have been involved. She describes in her book *Not Today Negativity!* how the "high-risk obstetrician office began to feel alarmingly like home."[1] She had begun feeling more at ease after she had a successful cerclage (a stitch to keep the cervix closed) placement at 12 weeks, and test after test and ultrasound after ultrasound revealed that all was going well with the pregnancy. While she had felt pelvic pain for several weeks and occasional contractions, approaching 23 weeks she felt safe enough to have her friends send out the shower invitations announcing her twin boys. Overall, she thought "everything was fine."[2]

There was nothing unusual leading up to the day of her routine visit with her high-risk doctor. The technician completed the ultrasound like every other time. Dr. Williams was not even concerned when she asked the technician, "How are things?," and got the answer, "The doctor will be right in."[3] Her doctor came and announced that one of her babies had died. She narrates her pain in her book: "I could not breathe. Searing pain ripped through my chest, and Niagara Falls tumbled down my face."[4] Just like that, the life of one of her children had ended.

Being pregnant with two or more babies places a mother and the babies at substantially higher risk. As cited by the *ACOG Practice Bulletin*, no. 231, risks to the babies include a higher likelihood of having abnormalities, stillbirth, and dying in the newborn period, mainly due to the increased risk associated with the baby being born preterm. Mothers face a higher risk of gestational diabetes (diabetes diagnosed in pregnancy), hypertensive disorders of pregnancy, anemia, hemorrhage, cesarean delivery, and postpartum depression, among others.[5]

The likelihood of having multiple births increases with age and use of artificial reproductive technology, factors that my grandmother and Dr. Williams had, respectively. However, for neither of them, as it is likely for most women, was it their motivation to place themselves at a higher risk for any condition; it was simply the universal motivation held by many women across the globe, the desire to parent children.

Before IVF pregnancies became more common, Black women in America were always more likely to give birth to twins as compared to White women. In 1980, the rate was 24.2 per 1,000 in Black women compared to 18.3 per White women.[6] This appears to be one of the true racial differences associated with being of African descent: Black women are more likely to have twins than White women. In fact, in 1999, 41% of the 2.8 million twins born were born in Africa, compared to 39% in Asia, 13% in America, 6% in Europe, and 0.5 % in Oceania.[7] While this was partly explained by the higher birth rate in Africa, the other explanation was that twin deliveries made up a higher proportion of the deliveries in the continent, almost twice the rate in Europe and three times the rate in Asia. The difference is not due to identical twins like my grandmother had but rather non-identical or fraternal twins, the type that is hereditary. In that time period, 52% of fraternal twins were born in the continent of Africa. That increased likelihood to have fraternal twins can be passed on genetically.

As the rates of twins and higher order multiple gestations increased among all women in America with the increasing use of fertility drugs and artificial reproductive technology and the increasing age of mothers,[8] the gap was essentially eliminated in 2012 to a rate of 36.8 per 1,000 (live births) in non-Hispanic (NH) White women compared to 36.9 per 1,000 for NH Black women. Recently, the differences have returned. In 2020, 112,437 babies were born in twin deliveries.[9] Overall, there was a 7% decline from 2019, a 2% decline for NH White women, a 3% decline for Hispanic women, but for NH Black women the rates were essentially the same, 40.9 per 1,000 births versus 40.7 per 1,000 births. The birth rates of multiples with three of more babies did decrease for all three groups of women. A potential explanation for the decrease in multiples was the stalling of assisted reproductive technology procedures for many months in 2020 due to the great deal of uncertainty surrounding the pandemic. Since Black women in America are less likely to benefit from these interventions and technologies, their twin birth rate did not decrease.

Even though Black women in America have higher rates of twin deliveries, which could potentially result in increased experience in the US healthcare system of caring for Black women with twins, they continue to have worse outcomes. I would be lying if I said I was surprised.

A secondary analysis of a multicenter study conducted by the Eunice Kennedy Shriver National Institute of Child Health and Human Development Maternal-Fetal Medicine Units Network evaluating the use of a medication that was hoped to prevent preterm birth in uncomplicated twin pregnancies was performed.[10] Women were enrolled in the study between April 2004 and February 2006. The study compared outcomes between women who self-identified as NH Black to those who self-identified as NH White. The analysis deliberately excluded pregnant women who had other factors that could increase their risk of additional complications, such as having any major chronic illness, carrying babies with major abnormalities, or other major twin-related complications. On average, Black women delivered a week and a half earlier than White women: at 33.6 weeks compared to 35.1 weeks—a significant span of time for a developing baby. Furthermore, for every prespecified gestational age cutoff (namely less than 28 weeks, less than 34 weeks, and less than 37 weeks), a higher proportion of Black women delivered preterm. They delivered earlier than White women across every gestational age; were more likely to be delivered for a complication, such as the baby not growing well in the womb; and their babies were more likely to die in the womb or as newborns.

Another study evaluating the rates of gestational diabetes mellitus (GDM) in twin pregnancy was performed analyzing the database from the Massachusetts General Hospital obstetric service between September 1, 1998, and December 31, 2006.[11] After statistical analysis to eliminate potential bias from other confounding factors, the rate of GDM was higher for twin pregnancies compared to singleton pregnancies (only one baby). African American women with twin pregnancies were more likely to have GDM than any other racial or ethnic group studied which included White, Latina and Asian women. What did this increased risk mean for the babies? The babies born to women with GDM had lower birthweights and were delivered at earlier gestational ages (34.3 weeks versus 36.1 weeks), which consequently increased their likelihood of other complications, including being admitted to the neonatal intensive care unit (NICU) and being in the hospital for more days.

The risks of twin pregnancies (and higher order multiples) are further increased if the babies share the same placenta and the same amniotic sac (monochorionic, monoamniotic twins) or if they have separate amniotic sacs but share the same placenta (monochorionic, diamniotic twins). Ideally, each baby has its own placenta and amniotic sac (dichorionic, diamniotic). While identical twins can involve any of those scenarios, fraternal twins, which have a higher prevalence in Black women, are always dichorionic, diamniotic because they develop from the fertilization of separate eggs from separate sperm rather than the splitting of one egg. Therefore, the increased risk that Black women face when they carry twin pregnancies is not due to a higher incidence of the riskiest types of twins.

Regardless of race, women with twin pregnancies need to be monitored closely, and the level of monitoring and needed intervention varies depending on which of the type twins they are. In the United States their care often involves high risk obstetricians like it did for Dr. Williams. However, there is a relatively low tech and inexpensive intervention that can help twin pregnancies be safer. A few years ago, Dr. William Goodnight and Dr. Roger Newman published an article advocating for optimizing nutrition for pregnant women carrying twins.[12] They discussed not only the importance of weight gain but also the timing of that weight gain, specifically weight gain by mid-pregnancy. They highlighted the importance of micronutrients as well as calorie composition in terms of calories from protein, carbohydrates, and fat. Among the research cited was The University of Michigan Multiples Clinic, a comprehensive prenatal program.[13] The program consisted of "(1) twice-monthly prenatal visits to a registered dietitian and nurse practitioner team in addition to the regular prenatal visits with the woman's primary care physician, (2) additional maternal education, (3) modification of maternal activity, (4) individualized dietary prescription, (5) multimineral supplementation, and (6) serial monitoring of nutritional status."[14] Women could be referred to the program by a healthcare team member or self-refer. Program mothers were older, less likely to smoke and more likely to have private or health maintenance organization (HMO) insurance compared to the mothers who were not in the program. Women in the program were significantly less likely to have their water break preterm (a factor highly correlated with delivering prematurely), less likely to delivery at less than 30 and 32 weeks, less likely to have a low-birthweight or a very low-birthweight baby, and less likely to have preeclampsia in addition to a lowering of the risk of multiple medical complications that especially affect premature newborns. Furthermore, the cost per twin was almost $15,000 less if their mother was in the program.

The only thing that I wondered after reading these findings was why this intervention was not implemented for pregnant women with twins or higher order multiples across the country? Although the study only had a small number of Black women, it is highly likely that this would be an effective intervention and easily justifiable by any insurance, including Medicaid, given the reduction in cost. Nevertheless, I certainly am not naive enough to think that this alone will close the gap in health disparities for Black women carrying multiple gestations. Even great nutrition will not be enough to reverse the negative impact of racism in its many forms on pregnancy of Black women, an impact likely magnified when a mother is carrying two or more babies. Nonetheless, it's a start.

About 8.5 weeks after her son Matthew died, Dr. Williams noticed that her frequent contractions were becoming more intense. She had to continue to carry her son, who had passed away, alongside his twin brother Mark who thankfully was progressing well. This is the case for every mother who carries multiples and loses one of them, while the other or others survive. As Dr. Williams describes, she had to "live with the heart-stopping fear of a similar outcome for Mark."[15]

Dr. Williams went to the nearby community hospital and had to be transferred by ambulance to a major Harvard hospital that could properly care for Mark if he needed to be delivered. When she was evaluated that was the decision that was made. The membranes that were holding in the amniotic fluid protecting Mark were bulging through her cervix, and due to the concern about a high risk of infection, delivery was recommended. It needed to be a cesarean section due to her prior fibroid surgery. At 31 weeks and 5 days, Mark was delivered. Dr. Oneeka Williams was able to hold him for a brief moment before he was taken to the NICU for specialized care. Her husband held Matthew as the priest blessed and baptized him.

My grandmother was lucky. She had the safe delivery of her twin daughters more than eighty years ago. However, the success of twin, and higher-order, pregnancies for Black women in America cannot be left to luck alone. It should be part of a concerted effort to ensure the safety of women pregnant with twins and higher-order multiples, especially when we already know they are at higher risks of complications. The level of support should be commensurate with the level of the risk.

CHAPTER 7

Preeclampsia/Hypertensive Disorders—
Too Common for Black Women

Preeclampsia is a condition I believe I care for well. I've cared for patients with the condition throughout my entire obstetric career, including patients who have developed serious life-threatening complications, and I believe I was well trained to identify preeclampsia quickly. It is a condition that, according to ACOG's definition, can develop in pregnancy usually after 20 weeks and involves new onset of high blood pressure and protein in the urine. However, women can have preeclampsia even without protein in the urine if they have other abnormalities usually detected by blood tests or if they have a headache that does not go away with medication or is not explained by other factors. If women have high blood pressure only, without the other signs or symptoms, and it starts after 20 weeks of pregnancy and returns to normal in the postpartum period, it is called gestational hypertension.[1] Sometimes a woman can come into pregnancy already having hypertension, and if she develops preeclampsia on top of that, it is called superimposed preeclampsia.[2]

Women who have preeclampsia can come to clinical care having already developed life-threatening symptoms or they can get worse in a short time after they get to the hospital. One of those complications is the development of seizures, called eclampsia.

As much as I consider myself good at caring for patients with preeclampsia, good does not mean perfect. I have had more than one patient over the course of my career present for clinical care with symptoms of preeclampsia and, while waiting for confirmatory lab tests or more blood pressure readings, they have seized. While I have chided myself when this happens, and tried to learn any lessons that I could, I avoided any self-flagellation in the moment. In the moment, I had to be laser focused. My objectives were clear: to protect the life of the mother; avoid any further seizures; and protect the life of the baby as soon as I have ensured that the mother was stable (not at any acute risk of dying). If I could possibly prevent it, no mother or baby was going to die on my watch. Since delivery is considered the cure for preeclampsia, if preeclampsia occurs while a woman is still pregnant, the plan of care does often involve delivery which could be either vaginal or a cesarean section. The route of delivery is a carefully considered decision that the obstetrician has to make. While in urgent life-threatening situations, as obstetricians, we can often call on other medical specialties to ensure that we are keeping the mother safe—for example, additional help from internal medicine physicians treating seizures if needed, anesthesiologist if she has breathing difficulties. However, the timing and route of delivery are up to us, the obstetricians, and in many settings it is a decision we make alone.

As obstetricians, our decisions can mean life or death. Did we make the diagnosis quickly enough? Did we start the treatment soon enough? Did we choose the right route of delivery, or did it lead to a complication that cost a mother her life? There may be times that by the time the mother comes into care it is already too late. Despite our best efforts and those of others, she cannot be saved.

The issue that arises especially when it comes to Black women in America and preeclampsia: one has to wonder which scenario cost a woman her life? Was it too late when the patient presented to care or were her clinicians too slow in diagnosing her and giving her the life-saving intervention she needed? Did they ignore her symptoms and tell her she should "take it easy" or that she was "stressing herself out?" Did they send her home when she should have been admitted to the hospital, and then when she returned it was too late? Those scenarios aren't just anecdotal stories of distraught family members. Preeclampsia/eclampsia and other hypertensive disorders are among the top reasons for any mother to die in the United States and worldwide.[3] However, in the United States, they are number one for Black women.[4] It appears that for the majority of Black women who have died from these conditions in America, it's not that they did not try to get the attention they needed in a timely manner rather it was the failure of the clinicians and/or the healthcare system to give them the timely care that they required.

In early 2017, the Maternal Mortality Review Committees published a report: "A View into their Critical Role."[5] The data was obtained through the partnership of four states (Colorado, Delaware, Georgia, and Ohio) working with the CDC and the CDC foundation. Included in their key findings was the fact that approximately 60% of the deaths were preventable. They attributed the causes of pregnancy-related deaths to three critical factors: (1) patients, which accounted for approximately 43%; (2) providers, another 35%; (3) and systems of care, 22%. (The facility itself accounted for less than 1%.) Despite citing patient factors to be the largest contributor, the study stated as follows: "While patient factors are the most common, these often reflect patient factors that are dependent on providers and systems of care, which becomes evident when put together with class and descriptions."[6] In that report, 41% of the women dying were non-Hispanic Black, 27.9% were non-Hispanic White, and 19.2% were Hispanic. In this report, preeclampsia and eclampsia tied with two other conditions—cardiomyopathy which I will discuss in chapter 15 and embolism described in chapter 14—for the leading cause of death among Black women.

For preeclampsia and eclampsia, the predominant critical factor was provider-related, which accounted for 62.2% of the total critical factors contributing to deaths. Of concern were the providers' assessment and knowledge. The analysis further uncovered where the providers were missing the mark: "misdiagnosis as the result of inadequate assessment and use of ineffective treatments."[7] In other words, the providers were failing to figure out the problem and giving the wrong treatment.

It turns out that the stories we continued to hear from distraught, predominantly Black, family members (since they bear the burden disproportionately) were true.

I have already discussed the role that implicit and explicit bias can play in compromising the care of Black pregnant women. Even when doctors know the right thing to do, their biases can interfere with them offering the correct treatment for Black women. They may think they mean well when they tell a woman to take it easy and not stress herself out. But all such advice is doing is leading to delay. Instead of figuring out what is causing the problem, the doctors blame the patient which in turn leads her to doubt herself. But clinician bias is only part of the problem.

I remember a patient whom I cared for during my private practice years in Jamaica. She was a lovely woman and a pleasure to take care of. She was mellow and easygoing. She was economically advantaged and had a supportive husband. She had no obvious risk factors entering her pregnancy, and to the best of my professional knowledge she was healthy. Yet several weeks before her due date I noticed that her blood pressure was getting elevated. Having enough suspicion about preeclampsia, I admitted her to the hospital for evaluation. Since her baby was preterm, if her diagnosis did not fall into the category of severe preeclampsia (currently described as preeclampsia with severe features), she could potentially continue the pregnancy with rest at home. With the help of trusted nursing staff, I monitored her for a few days in the community hospital where I delivered. She was doing well.

The nurses felt that she could return home. I saw her one evening, but decided I would keep her one more night and reevaluate her laboratory tests in the morning. The following morning her blood pressures started to creep up and her lab tests showed some slight abnormalities. She continued to look well and did not show any other visible signs or symptoms that her condition was worsening. But I knew the changes were not a good sign. I promptly arranged transfer to the University hospital—the only facility available to care for a preterm baby of that gestation. I noted that the admitting physician seemed to doubt the urgency of the situation that I was conveying, but fortunately she accepted the transfer. The transfer was not immediate. I repeated the patient's laboratory test while she waited. After she was transferred to the University hospital, a less than thirty-minute ambulance ride, I continued to check in with the staff on duty about the timing of the delivery. I felt that it had become urgent. When the last set of laboratory tests returned, my fears were confirmed and I promptly called the hospital.

The patient's labs had worsened, and she had developed severe thrombocytopenia: her platelets, which are essential for blood clotting and preventing life-threatening bleeding, had dropped precipitously.

It was part of HELLP (hemolysis, elevated liver enzymes, low platelet count) syndrome, a known complication of preeclampsia. My call coincided with the hospital's receipt of critical lab information they had also collected. They were taking the patient to the operating room immediately to deliver the baby, only a few hours after I had seen her that morning. Fortunately, both mother and baby did well and made an excellent recovery. The patient resumed her care with me in the postpartum period.

To what did I attribute my decision to keep her that extra night—a decision that might have been life-saving? Was it my experience and training? Was it divine intervention? I think it was both. I was grateful, and humbly realized that if I had gone the other way, even though there was reasonably evidence that I could have, she may not have made it. This leads me to the other reason why the care of women, and Black women in particular, may be compromised when they receive a diagnosis of preeclampsia or another hypertensive disorder of pregnancy.

Could it be that some clinicians who deliver maternal care are unable to properly recognize one of the major conditions that cause women to die? I have discussed aspects of this in other chapters and will raise some additional insights here. The reasons might include some significant shifts of healthcare delivery in the United States. Between 2004 and 2014, some 179 hospitals lost their ability to provide obstetric care to women.[8] The implication of this is that if a pregnant woman with one of these life-threatening conditions needs emergency care at one of those facilities, she is not likely to be seen by an obstetrician or allied health professional trained to deliver such care, or even a physician.

I believe that too many members of the current workforce are inadequately trained to diagnose and care for medical problems that pregnant women face. I believe this is related to the ever-expanding categories of providers in the US healthcare system, the shortage of physicians, and the inconsistency of training of clinicals, including advanced-practice practitioners (APPs).

The changes in the healthcare system have another significant consequence: physician burnout. At least half of obstetricians and gynecologists experience burnout.[9] The consequence of this problem is that, despite being adequately trained, an obstetrician suffering from burnout is more likely to make a medical error. Another consequence is the departure of some well-trained obstetricians from the field alto-gether, further compromising the workforce delivering care to preg-nant women. This fact highlights the need for improved education of all clinicians who deliver obstetric care, including emergency room clinicians, and assurance that these clinicians exhibit core competen-cies based on the known factors that drive the maternal morbidity and mortality rates. Urgent attention also needs to be directed at measures to reduce physician burnout.

During the pandemic I read the tragic story of the death of Dr. Chaniece Wallace, a fourth-year pediatric resident at the Indiana University School of Medicine,[10] from complications of preeclampsia four days after her daughter was born via emergency cesarean section. My mind was flooded with questions: Did the doctors diagnose her too late, or did she present to care too late? Did they act quickly enough, or did they miss important clues? Or was her death inevitable despite them doing everything they could? None of us are God, but do we do the best that we were trained to do for all our patients? Sadly, the answer is no.

Among Dr. Wallace's complications was a "ruptured liver"—a known, but rare and severe, complication of preeclampsia/eclampsia and/or HELLP syndrome. "Ruptured liver" can refer to spontaneous rupture of a subcapsular liver hematoma (collection of blood between the liver and a layer of tissue surrounding it) or of the liver itself. It is a rare incident occurring in 1 in 40,000 to 1 in 250,000 deliveries and in about 1% to less than 2% of the cases with HELLP syndrome.[11]

I remember one such case in my entire professional career, including my four years of residency training. It was in a Latina woman. I was still in training and thankfully not in charge, only a part of the team. However, I still remember how impressed I was with the African American general surgeon who went to the operating room with our obstetric team. He was confident and ready to do anything it would take to save our patient's life. He was able to control the bleeding quickly, and our patient recovered well without having to undergo any major surgery on her liver. Again, I was not really sure if our success was related to our timely intervention or divine intervention. Here, too, I think it was both.

Saving any woman who has developed preeclampsia depends on timely diagnosis and treatment. While there are new developments on the way to help us with our diagnosis, we have to be well trained on how to diagnose and treat the condition promptly, not just in Black women, but not excluding Black women. While preeclampsia is not a Black woman's disease, it is clear that implicit, and potentially explicit, bias is interfering with the care that Black women receive. National and statewide policy must ensure that the hospitals where reproductive-age women seek care have adequately trained and culturally sensitive clinicians who can, at the minimum, stabilize the patients until they can get to a more specialized facility. Their decision-making can be enhanced by prompt and easily obtainable obstetric support, even in the telemedicine format combined with adequate training for APPs that they know what urgent interventions to do and when to seek help and support.

APPs and other clinicians should have the ability to contact obstetricians anytime they need their support. Given the time zone differences, it is not inconceivable that a call placed at 3:00 a.m. EST may be answered by a physician at midnight PST, minimizing the stress of any supporting obstetrician, especially with the dwindling obstetric workforce. Having done night shifts for most of my obstetric career, a midnight support call when I might be just going to sleep is much less taxing than a 3:00 a.m. call which is more likely to disrupt a deep sleep.

I am confident that a vast number of obstetricians, if fairly compensated, could make themselves available to offer training to APPs, either remotely or in person, as circumstances permit. Many might be willing to offer urgent telemedicine support if they are shielded from unreasonable liability risks.

In addition, this type of support can help with key life-saving intervention decisions for the other life-threatening obstetric complications. Why do Black women disproportionately die from hypertensive disorders of pregnancy? Is it just related to the fact that they are less likely to be diagnosed and treated in a timely manner or do they develop these conditions more often, or both?

It is both. In a study evaluating hypertensive disorders among women who have never given birth before, Black women are more likely to have chronic hypertension before they get pregnant and more likely to develop mild, severe, or superimposed preeclampsia,[12] despite being younger than the average age of women studied, 22.7 years old compared to an average age of 26.4 for White women. Other women in the study included Hispanic women, Asian/Pacific Islanders, and multiracial or other races. Only 18% of Black women were married, compared to 74% of White women and 84.3% of Asian/Pacific Islanders. While Black women were more likely to have a higher body mass index (BMI, a marker of obesity), their average pre-pregnancy BMI was only 26.1, which is well below the obesity range of 30. The average number for White women was 24.1. However, Black women were less likely to smoke than White women. Interestingly, Asian/Pacific Islanders were more likely than even White women to have a normal blood pressure throughout pregnancy and least likely to develop mild preeclampsia compared to all the groups of women studies.

As for the reasons Black women in America are more likely to develop hypertensive disorders of pregnancy, I have already discussed the effects of racism on inducing chronic illnesses at younger ages in Black women. Chronic illnesses include hypertension. What about pregnancy itself, when the woman starts pregnancy without any hypertensive disease?

A study published in 2021 evaluated data from just over 6,000 women who delivered at Boston Medical Center (the largest safety net hospital in Boston) between October 1, 1998 and February 15, 2016 (the Boston Birth Cohort). It found that non-Hispanic Black women who were not born in America had a 26% lower risk of preeclampsia than Black women who were born in America. In fact, if foreign-born Black women lived in the United States for less than ten years, they were 38% less likely to develop preeclampsia, but this decreased risk disappeared if they lived in America for more than ten years.[13] In an earlier analysis of the data findings, one of the study authors commented about the waning of the "healthy immigrant effect" over time. The healthy immigrant effect refers to immigrants being healthier when they come to the United States.[14] However, this waning over time did not occur for White or Hispanic women. Their risk of preeclampsia did not get worse if they stayed in the United States more than ten years. Furthermore, there was no difference in the rates of preeclampsia for White and Hispanic women whether or not they were born in the United States despite the fact that US-born of all the groups studies, White, Black and Hispanic had more risk factors for cardiovascular disease than their non-US-born counterparts.

This finding may not come as a surprise to Dr. Oneeka Williams, (who I spoke about in chapter 6), a urologic surgeon, Medical Director, and award-winning author living in Massachusetts, who despite being born outside the United States faced a myriad of pregnancy-related complications, including a hypertensive disorder, which developed 3 weeks after she gave birth to her first child, about twenty years after she came to the United States to attend Johns Hopkins University. Although she was not able to name it fifteen years ago, when her son was born, she now fully believes that her outcomes were affected by the stress that racism had placed on her health and the health of her pregnancy.

How can we better diagnose women so we can intervene in time? Exciting new technology may be one of the keys. An experimental blood test had shown promise in predicting preeclampsia, and while it might be only able to identify three quarters of cases of preeclampsia, it is still better than any available test today.[15]

While we wait for this technology to be fully developed, we still need to capitalize on any tools we already have. As Benjamin Franklin once said, an ounce of prevention is better than a pound of cure.[16] Can preeclampsia be prevented?

Maybe not for every woman, but we certainly have evidence that we can reduce the risk. Low-dose aspirin has been recommended as an effective treatment to reduce the risk of preeclampsia in women who are at high risk for the disease and who can safely use this treatment.[17] For the best efficacy, ACOG recommends that it be started before 16 weeks of pregnancy. I'll state the obvious: we can't know what we don't know. Healthcare-delivery systems across the country need to ensure that their clinicians are aware of this intervention and in which patients the therapy needs to be implemented. Because of the multiple inequities Black women face, many will fit the category for being "at high risk." Electronic Medical Records (EMRs) are used extensively across the United States. According to data compiled by the CDC, approximately 90% of office-based physicians use EMRs.[18] With technology being advanced as it is, prompts should be developed to alert clinicians of this recommended treatment when the relevant risk factors are documented in the chart. While they may help patients, EMRs have placed extensive burdens on clinicians: EMR technology should be used to increase clinician support, rather than increase their workload.[19] While low-dose aspirin in pregnant women did not appear to be harmful in the studies, medication invariably is not risk-free and there may be patients who are concerned about risks. Are there other prevention options that could be essentially risk-free? In fact, there are.

A study evaluating Norwegian women, who were giving birth for the first time, demonstrated a reduced risk of preeclampsia in women who reported that they had a high intake of vegetables and fruit, including berries, in their diet, which also consisted of rice, vegetable oils, including olive oil, and poultry.[20] On the other hand, women who reported that they were more likely to eat a lot of processed foods, including sausages, hamburgers, white bread, salty snacks, sugar-sweetened drinks, and sweets, had an increased risk of preeclampsia. This questionnaire was specifically designed to get information on women's dietary habits during the first 4–5 months of pregnancy, and it was completed by the time the women were about 22 weeks pregnant.

A meta-analysis, which cited the Norwegian study, also showed a reduced risk of preeclampsia in women who received interventions aimed at improving their diet which sometimes included healthy dietary advice by a nutritionist or the implementation of a cholesterol-lowering diet.[21] However, many of the studies in the meta-analysis focused on targeting women with gestational diabetes. Nevertheless, a key component of effective interventions was initiation in the first trimester.

Do these findings apply to American women and specifically Black women in America? Yes, they do. Another study looking at the Boston Birth Cohort supported the use of a Mediterranean diet in reducing the risk of preeclampsia among women.[22] Specifically, the authors created a Mediterranean-style diet score (MSDS) based on information derived from a food-frequency questionnaire that the women were given 24 to 72 hours after delivery. The authors organized the scores into three categories (tertiles), with the third tertile correlating with the diets that most closely matched the Mediterranean-style diet. They found a decreased risk of preeclampsia with improved diet, even after excluding women who entered pregnancy with diabetes or hypertension. In further analysis, specifically considering Black women, the authors found that, statistically, Black women appeared to benefit the most from the Mediterranean-style diet.

The research suggests very important strategies to reduce the rates of hypertensive disorders in Black pregnant women. Reproductive-aged Black women should receive continuing education on the impact of a healthy diet that emphasizes the benefits not only for their own health but also that of their baby. Early entry into prenatal care should be facilitated, and continued dietary advice and support should be given. While nutrition-counseling support may be sufficient for more affluent Black women, low-income Black women may need additional support in procuring healthy foods, particularly if they live in food deserts, a problem which plagues many Black communities. Getting the food might not be the only problem: with increasing reliance on fast foods, younger generations of Black women may be losing important skills in food preparation, or if they do have the skills, they are restricted to the preparation of poorer quality diets.

A few years ago, when I held a leadership position at Baltimore Medical System, a federally qualified health center (FQHC) in Baltimore, I wanted to encourage my staff to eat more healthily. Aware that some of them were excellent cooks, I decided to launch a competition to prepare a tasty plant-based meal. No one entered. I questioned one of my African American staff members who, I knew, had outstanding skills, having had the pleasure to taste her food at other events.

"Aren't you going to enter?" I asked.

"Dr. Rainford, you said no meat. I'm not going to do that." She had no intention of entering a cooking competition that did not allow her to include meat.

I abandoned my well-intentioned, but obviously ill-informed, effort. I designed a competition to try to improve the health of my team without considering their priorities. Courses could be designed from the expanding domain of culinary medicine[23] to educate pregnant women to prepare healthier meals with careful consideration of cultural norms. Furthermore, as I have discussed in many chapters including chapters 5 and 6, reducing the risk of preeclampsia is not the only way that pregnant women can benefit from a healthy diet.

We cannot prevent preeclampsia or every hypertensive disorder in every Black pregnant woman, or in pregnant women in general. We cannot save or prevent complications in every pregnant woman, even if we are good, or even great, physicians or midwives. But, as we think about Dr. Chaniece Wallace and all those many women who have died or suffered from these conditions, the question we need to continually ask in any capacity we serve, whether directly in healthcare or not, is, are we doing everything we can to protect and save pregnant women. If we are being honest with ourselves, the answer too often is we are not.

CHAPTER 8

Stillbirth—The Searing Pain of Loss and Why Black Women Suffer More

I tried to comfort her each time I stepped into her room, but it seemed of little use. I could hear her cries of anguish every time I walked by. She was supported by many loving family members, but it didn't seem to help. She had lost her baby at about 28 weeks. If we had been able to predict and deliver her baby early, her premature baby could have had a chance at survival. I met Mrs. Anderson,* an African American woman in her thirties, during my residency. I was on an obstetric rotation at one of our partner hospitals and she was diagnosed with a stillbirth. Her baby had died in the womb, and she had been admitted to the hospital to induce labor, the common method used to deliver stillbirths at that gestation.

Labor induction can be an arduous process for any pregnant person. Women sometimes receive multiple doses of medications to force their body to have uterine contractions and go into labor. It can sometimes take several days, and often mothers find the long process tiring and sometimes frustrating. But at least most people who undergo an induction have the birth of their babies to look forward to. This is not true for a mother with a stillbirth. The whole process is just pain. We do our best to ease it with medication, but medication does not ease grief. Nothing eased Mrs. Anderson's pain: not the kind words of the doctors and nurses, not the comfort of all the family members who were in the room, not the heartfelt prayers.

A labor-and-delivery room is larger than a typical hospital room. It often has special finishing touches, such as wood veneer on the cabinet doors, and other efforts to make it appear more homey. I recall multiple family members being present. I recall the buzz of conversation. I recall food being shared. I recall a feeling of warmth when I entered. I doubt Mrs. Anderson felt that warmth. She had lost her baby; I think it was her only child. I have diagnosed other stillbirths since then, and it is always difficult news to deliver, but I will never forget Mrs. Anderson. She was one of my first patients with a stillbirth, and the depth of her grief touched me to the core.

Stillbirth is the loss of a baby after 20 weeks of pregnancy; and for every 160 births, one will be stillborn.[1] Black women are more than twice as likely to have a stillbirth than White or Hispanic women,[2] per data from the National Vital Statistics Reports the 2019 rates being 10.4 per 1,000 live births compared to 4.71 for White women.[3] In general, rates of stillbirths are higher for women between the ages of fifteen and nineteen, and increase progressively for women thirty-five and older. For Black women, the lowest rates occur when they are in their twenties but get worse if they have their babies any younger or any older. The sad reality is that even the lowest rates for Black women are higher than the worst rates for White women. Furthermore, in some states the rates of stillbirth for Black babies are even higher. During the period 2015–2017, in the state of New Jersey, for every 1,000 Black babies born alive, 17 Black babies were born dead.[4] The question is why?

First, it is important to understand the causes of stillbirth and how they differ for Black women. Again referencing the National Vital Statistics Reports between 30% and 33% of the time we don't know the cause of stillbirth, regardless of the race of the mother.[5] We as obstetricians deliver a baby that looks normal to us, and sometimes despite a battery of tests for both the mother and the baby, we can't pinpoint the cause. For both Black and White women, the next most common cause—about a quarter of stillbirths—is problems with the placenta, cord, and/or membranes. For the remaining 40% of stillbirths, the reasons look a little different. For Black women, almost 30% of the time the cause is attributed to two categories, pregnancy-related maternal complications, or maternal conditions not related to the pregnancy. For White women this is less than 20%. Maternal conditions include conditions that existed prior to pregnancy, for example high blood pressure, kidney disease, or lupus and complications are those that happen to the mother during the pregnancy, many of which are mentioned throughout this book.

Racism negatively impacts the health of Black women not only by accelerating their biological aging, increasing their risk of chronic diseases, causing them to die prematurely, and affecting their pregnancies, but it appears to be killing their babies even before they can be born. In 2009, the United States National Institutes of Health (NIH) published a study which involved an extensive evaluation of the stillbirths that took place in 2001 and 2002.[6] Thirty-six states were selected because they had sufficient data entry for certain criteria including Hispanic ethnicity, delivery method, and prenatal care. At every gestational age, Black women were more likely to have stillbirths than White or Hispanic women. At that time, Black women were overall twice as likely to have a stillbirth. The disparity was the greatest between 20 and 23 weeks, and then decreasing except for a slight increase at 41 weeks. From 20 to 27 weeks of pregnancy, the biggest risk of a baby dying in the womb was due to pregnancy-related complications, such as a woman's water breaking early or a woman developing a hypertension-related problem during her pregnancy. For women who lost their babies at full term, their prior medical conditions posed the greatest risk. Additionally, the study showed that a Black woman was between one and a half to two times as likely as a White woman to lose her baby between 39 and 41 weeks, gestations when most babies can survive outside the womb without any medical support. Despite this disparity, Black women were *less* likely to be induced than White women. Induction is the same process that they would likely have to undergo to get out a dead baby—a baby that they will never get to know. Why is induction not being used more often to allow Black women to have a baby that they will have the joy of knowing? Even when certain medical conditions could signal to the obstetrician that labor should probably be induced, some Black mothers are still not getting the procedure in time to save their babies.

While education protected White women against stillbirth, it did little to protect Black women. If a White woman had more than twelve years of education, she was 30% less likely to have a stillbirth, but the same level of education in Black women only offered minimal benefit. Furthermore, as the authors of the study chose to highlight, the

Black–White disparity was even larger for Black women with higher education. I was fascinated to see that, even at the time the study was published, the authors were able to cite prior research showing that educational status was not protecting the infants of Black women and that the possible implications of racism had already been recognized. Specifically, a study published in 1998 in the *American Journal of Public Health* failed to show any substantial protective effect of maternal education on the infant mortality rate for Black women, despite a 20% risk reduction for White women.[7] In 2005, Giscombe and Lobel offered a more detailed analysis of the how stress and racism deleteriously affected the pregnancy outcomes of African American women.[8]

A few years later, some of the same NIH researchers decided to dig deeper. Recognizing that stress, including that of racial discrimination, likely had a negative impact on the pregnancy outcome of Black women, they examined how certain life events in the twelve months prior to delivery impacted the stillbirth rate.[9] Significant life events (SLEs) were grouped into four factors: financial, emotional, traumatic, and partner-related events. Financial SLEs included having a husband or partner without a job, losing a job, or having a lot of bills that could not be paid. Emotional SLEs included moving to a new address, being homeless, having a husband or partner who went to jail or being jailed themselves, traumatic events including having a close family member who was sick or had to go to the hospital or someone very close dying. Partner-related events included being separated or divorced from a partner, arguing with a partner more than usual, husband or partner not wanting them to be pregnant, being in a physical fight, or having someone very close with drinking or drugs problems. The risk of stillbirth increased incrementally with the number of SLEs reported. Black women were both more likely to have SLEs than White women (except for traumatic events) and to have multiple SLEs compared to White women. Inability to pay bills was significantly associated with more stillbirths for both Blacks and Whites.

Interestingly, although Black women were more than twice as likely as White women to have a partner in jail or to be in jail themselves, or to be separated or divorced from their partner, these events in isolation did not appear to affect the stillbirth rates of Black women. Rather, it was the fact that they were more likely to have any SLE, and the sheer frequency of SLEs that Black women experienced, that seemed to create the disparity.

How can we fix this? We cannot prevent all stillbirths, but the existing disparities make clear that this is yet another example of our society failing Black women and their babies.

Some interventions are relatively easy to implement. As clinicians, given the evidence that induction does not increase the C-section risk in women giving birth for the first time,[10] we should be as generous with offering 39-week inductions to our Black patients as we are to our White patients. We should ensure that Black mothers with other medical conditions are among the top of the list for being offered induction or delivery at 39 weeks of pregnancy or earlier if their condition merits. Delivery planning should be a part of an ongoing conversation with our patients during the pregnancy so that they can have a clear understanding of the motivations.

Furthermore, we need to ensure that Black women receive equitable prenatal care. If they have medical conditions, they need to be prescribed timely treatments and interventions that meet recognized standards of care. Any barriers to accessing care need to be recognized and addressed. But this is not the only thing we can do.

In low-income countries, where mothers suffer from malnutrition due to inadequate calorie intake, studies have shown that supplementing their diet with balanced energy protein reduces the risk of stillbirth.[11] These supplements are food-based with less than 25% of the total energy content coming from proteins. For example, in Gambia, the supplement contained nuts, nut oil, rice flour, and sugar. The risk for African American women is not usually inadequate calorie intake but rather poor-quality diet. Furthermore, recent studies have shown the correlation with a poor-quality diet and poor growth of the baby in the womb.[12] ACOG, in their Obstetric Care Consensus (a series of documents jointly developed with the Society for Maternal-Fetal Medicine) related to the management of stillbirth, describes fetal growth restriction (poor fetal growth) as "associated with a significant increase in the risk of stillbirth."[13] Regardless of the weight or body size of the mother, her diet might still lack the necessary components to ensure that her baby's growth is healthy. Animal research has even shown that a typical American diet can lead to stillbirth.[14] Furthermore, studies have already shown that obesity,[15] a condition more prevalent among Black women in America, is associated with stillbirth.

Can we do more to support healthy eating for Black pregnant women? To be clear, "support" means more than giving them a brochure, without ensuring that they can access the food both financially and logistically. During my time as a medical director for two of the centers of Baltimore Medical System, Hungry Harvest (an organization dedicated to decreasing the waste of fruits and vegetables and making them available at a lower cost) established a location on the parking lot outside our building. I was grateful for the initiative, but I realized that for some of our patients it may still not be enough. The cost may be prohibitive, or they may simply lack the knowledge to prepare the foods in a tasty, healthy manner. Can additional support be given to these women? The American College of Lifestyle Medicine through the HEAL (Health Equity Achieved through Lifestyle Medicine) initiative has been working on interventions to bridge the gap between the Black and White communities. However, more help is needed as these initiatives are not yet focused on Black pregnant women. Black women with higher incomes may simply need information about one of the many food services offering healthy meal kits which can be prepared quickly, or culturally sensitive instructions on preparing healthy meals. If government spending cannot yet be approved for these initiatives, can philanthropy meet this need?

Erika Ota, a midwife and professor based in Japan, in collaboration with other researchers recently published a comprehensive review of interventions to prevent stillbirths.[16] In addition to the dietary interventions discussed above, she reported on other initiatives that have been proven to be beneficial to reduce stillbirths. Among the effective interventions were midwife-led models of care which not only decreased overall loss of babies in the womb but specifically reduced stillbirths before 24 weeks.[17] While these studies were done outside the United States, they were done in other developed countries such as Australia, Canada, Ireland, and the United Kingdom, all of which have better maternal mortality rates than the United States and equal or better stillbirth rates compared to the United States. I was particularly impressed by the finding of reduced stillbirths before 24 weeks, gestations where Black women experience the worse health disparities.

It is time to double down on the government and NGO efforts to encourage the training of midwives to include an emphasis on educating Black midwives and others who are particularly interested in supporting Black mothers. Scholarships could be tied to an obligation to support Black communities in a similar manner to that of the National Health Service Corps (NHSC) which currently supports healthcare providers who desire to serve in medically underserved communities. I have noticed outstanding commitment and dedication of the scholars I have worked with in the past, and I believe that having more of these programs will lead to a greater number of outstanding clinicians who are willing to not only support health of Black women but also expand the capacity to care for all women in America.

Another area that I believe is worth investigating further is community-based interventions. Although studies on these types of interventions were mainly done in developing countries,[18] reductions in stillbirth rates were seen for initiatives particularly if they involved community mobilization and home visits during pregnancy. Specific initiatives involved training female health workers who were members of the community and establishing volunteer community health committees.[19] During the intervention, they visited pregnant women in their homes. We should empower low-income urban or rural Black communities in a similar manner.

But what of highly educated, high-income Black women? We already know that they are at least as vulnerable to stillbirths as low-income Black women, so what can we do to help? One component of the success of the community-based programs were home visits. Let's adapt this insight to the digital age. Given the abundance of telemedicine platforms, one or several can be used to supplement the care of Black women with telemedicine visits. Due to the current state of healthcare, office visits are often rushed, and patients often see a different clinician on every visit. Large employers should provide financial coverage for these additional remote visits with obstetricians or midwives as an additional resource to answer questions. I believe an intervention will be most efficacious if, during those visits, women can establish continuity with the same remote clinician throughout the pregnancy; however, it should be clear to the patients that these visits are supplemental, and not a substitute for their primary OB/GYN care. The telemedicine-support clinicians should have the appropriate training to ensure they understand the unique needs of their Black patients.

Such interventions require investment so that they can be studied and evaluated scientifically. Effective interventions need to be documented and shared and that work needs to be expanded. The financial benefits need to be detailed so that initiatives can be sustained. Too often I hear stories of successful interventions that fell by the wayside due to loss of funding or interest.

None of these initiatives are suggested as an alternative to standards of care recognized by expert maternal care bodies, but rather as a supplement. Fortunately, the overall stillbirth rates have been trending downward in the United States; nonetheless, the large disparity for Black women remains. I am also confident that the lessons learned can be applied to decrease the stillbirth rate in other communities that suffer disparities.

I never learned what happened to Mrs. Anderson. I will never know whether she went on to give birth to a healthy child or children. I will never know what steps she had to take to move beyond her grief, or whether the loss has continued to have a strong hold on her throughout her life. Wanda Irving, Dr. Shalon Irving's mother, once told me "unless you walked in those shoes, you really, really do not understand what it means to lose a child. And it's not just an adult child, but any child."[20]

"The grief doesn't end; it may be easier to get through it, but you never get over it."[21]

As bystanders, we might think that such overwhelming grief affects only mothers who have lost children they were able to see alive; but when I think of Mrs. Anderson, I believe Mrs. Wanda Irving's words ring no less true for mothers of stillborn children.

CHAPTER 9

Low Birthweight Babies—What's in a Number?

I started having my children when I was over the age of thirty-five. It was not a deliberate decision. Having completed my obstetrics and gynecology training a couple of years before I turned thirty, I was thoroughly educated on the increased complications that women and babies could face when a woman of advanced maternal age (the medical term for pregnant women aged thirty-five and over) became pregnant. While I had some comfort in the fact that my maternal grandmother had three successful pregnancies over the age of thirty-five, the last being twins, as I've described, I fretted as the years went by, as I got older and older, and I had not met the person I wanted to marry. Perhaps influenced by my religion, my career choice, and the family structure I grew up in, I never wanted to parent alone, so I waited.

Despite the age-related risk, I had normal pregnancies. Apart from a brief scare, the possibility of gestational diabetes, and some initially concerning ultrasound findings during my first pregnancy with my son, everything went well. After getting a higher-than-normal value on the one-hour glucose-tolerance screening, a standard for most pregnant women, I made adjustments to improve my diet and passed the three-hour test. My son had ultrasound findings which were a bit concerning, but after a follow-up ultrasound by the high-risk-pregnancy doctor, everything turned out to be fine.

My pregnancies went so well, in fact, that the weights of my children were only two ounces apart. My son was born at about 39.5 weeks, and he weighed seven pounds and six ounces, and my daughter, who was born at exactly 39 weeks, weighed 7 pounds and 3.8 ounces. They were normal, average-weight babies.[1] Over the years, as I have delivered babies, that's one of the most common questions I get from new parents: How much does the baby weigh?

I took the birthweights of my children for granted. At that time, I didn't know that babies of US-born Black women had on average lower birthweights that those of US-born White women. I did not realize how my parents' decision to leave New York and raise me in Jamaica, and even my decision to return to Jamaica in my early thirties, before I got married, had potentially not only protected me from many pregnancy complications but also protected the birthweights of my children. I did not know that the birthweights of my children could be associated with lifelong health and economic risks. Two researchers examined the long-term effects of low birthweights (LBWs) using a nationally representative sample of the US population. They found that, compared to their normal-birthweight siblings, low-birthweight children were less likely to be in "very good" or "excellent" health in childhood, scored less well on school tests, and were more likely to drop out of high school. Furthermore, low-birthweight children were more likely than their siblings to have health problems from ages thirty-seven to fifty-two, and in their thirties and forties their health was equivalent to the health of someone twelve years older. There was also an effect on their annual earnings: it lagged 10 to 22% behind other adults in their respective age group.[2] Chronic diseases associated with low birthweight include obesity, coronary heart disease, and chronic kidney disease.[3]

As I had mentioned in the introduction, I was often told that the disparities between Black and White women were blamed on socioeconomic status. When researchers realized that socioeconomic status did not protect Black women, they started to blame it on the genetic makeup.

In the 1990s, two physician researchers, Dr. Richard David and Dr. James Collins, decided to put that theory to the test.[4] They hypothesized that since it is estimated that US Black people derived three quarters of their genetic heritage from West Africans and the rest from Europeans, the babies with "pure" West African origin should be smaller than US-born Black babies who were already known to be smaller than White babies. They specifically compared the birthweights of babies of

US-born Black women to the birthweights of US-born babies of women who were born in one of the seventeen countries in the regions where African slaves originated from, and to the babies of US-born White women. The sample consisted of babies born in Illinois between 1980 and 1995. The researchers found quite the opposite. The average birthweight of a White baby was 3,446 grams (approximately 7 pounds, 9.6 ounces). The average weight of the baby of an African-born Black woman was 3,333 grams (7 pounds 5.6 ounces—close to the weights of my two children) and the average weight of a baby of a US-born Black woman was 3,089 grams (6 pounds 13 ounces). The distribution of the birthweights of babies of African-born Black women closely resembled that of babies of White women: The incidence of low birthweight (weight less than 2,500 grams) was 13.2% among infants of US-born Black women and 7.1% among infants of African-born Black women, as compared with 4.3% among infants of US-born White women (relative risks, 3.1 and 1.6, respectively). The only birthweights that were similar for both African-born and US-born Black women were very-low-birthweight (VLBW) babies (weighing less than 1,500 grams).

Clearly, the African genes are not the reason why there is such a disparity in the birthweights between the babies of US-born Black and White women.

In a follow-up study, the same two authors, partnered with another researcher, and compared the birthweights for Caribbean-born Black women and US-born Black women.[5] The Caribbean-born Black women were mainly from Jamaica (37%), Haiti (27%), and Belize (11%). Caribbean-born Black women share the legacy of slavery, like US-born Black women, and depending on the country may have varying levels of European influence in the gene pool.[6] The distribution of the weights of babies of Caribbean-born Black mothers again closely matched those of babies of US-born White mothers, and differed from the birthweights of the babies of US-born Black mothers. However, the average weights were not reported in this study. While the rates of VLBW babies were again comparable between Caribbean- and US-born Black women, the moderately-low-birthweight (MBLW) babies (1,500–2,499 grams) were 10% for the babies of US-born Black women, compared to 6% for Caribbean-born Black women and 4% for US-born White women. The article shared two additional important pieces of information. Citing other studies, the authors noted that there is no difference in rates of LBW between US-born and foreign-born White women. Based on their own study, they noted that if the maternal risk factors for White mothers decreased, these mothers were less likely to give birth to VLBW babies. This protection was not present for Black mothers, whether US- or Caribbean-born. Whether Black mothers had more than twelve years of education, whether they were married, whether they had adequate prenatal care, and whether their babies' fathers had more than twelve years of education, the disparity remained. The Black–White disparity was greater if the mother had fewer risk factors.

Linda Villarosa, former executive editor of Essence magazine, an associate professor, and a New York Times Magazine contributor, is personally aware of the disparities. Despite her stellar educational background, excellent health and health insurance she too gave birth to a 4-pound 13-ounce (2,183 grams) low birthweight baby when her daughter had to be delivered one month before her due date due to intrauterine growth restriction (IUGR, or poor growth in the uterus).[7] She further chronicles the effects of racism on the health of Americans in her book *Under the Skin*.[8] There are a number of behaviors that can affect the growth of babies in the womb, such as smoking, drinking, drug abuse, not eating adequately to gain enough weight. There are other factors, such as an infection or preexisting medical conditions, for example hypertension or diabetes.[9] Or, as in the case of Linda Villarosa, the baby's low weight could be due solely to the adverse effects that racism can have on a Black woman's body before and during her pregnancy.

How quickly does racism affect the birthweight advantage of foreign-born Black women? Dr. Collins and Dr. David partnered with another colleague to examine this factor.[10] They linked the birthweight data of female babies born in Illinois between 1989 and 1991 (generation 3) to mothers also born in Illinois between 1956 and 1975 (generation 2). The maternal grandmothers were generation 1. They found that for generation-1 US- and European-born White mothers, their babies got bigger by generation 3. The generation-3 babies of US-born White mothers were 65 grams heavier than the babies of the generation-2 mothers. The generation-3 babies were 45 grams heavier for generation-1 European-born White women. The rate of MLBW was 10%

lower for generation-3 versus generation-2 US-born White mothers. There was no difference in the rate of MLBW for European-born White women across the generations, and the numbers of VLBW were too few for an estimate. Even for US-born Black women, there was an increase in birthweight between generation 2 and generation 3, but only 17 grams, while the rate of MLBW was the same and there was a threefold increase of VLBW. This was not the case for foreign-born Black mothers. The data suggested that the birthweights of generation 3 were 57 grams lower than generation-2, and the babies were 40% more likely to be MLBW. Possibly related to the low numbers in the sample of foreign-born Black women (104), the decrease in birthweights did not reach statistical significance, so it is possible that the decrease was due to chance.

Another pair of researchers from Princeton University decided to put the findings to the test.[11] This time, they examined the birth-weight data for women in Florida, given the high concentration of Caribbean-born Black immigrants in the state. They also wanted to see how the findings compared to the Hispanic immigrant populations. They looked at Florida birth records between 1971 and 2015. Their G1, or grandmother generation, were women who gave birth between 1971 and 1995; the G2, or mother generation, were born during those years; and the G3, or the generations of daughters of G2, were born between 1989 and 2015. The foreign-born White women were mainly from Canada and Europe; the Hispanic-born women were mainly from Cuba or Mexico; and the Caribbean-born Black women were mainly from Jamaica and Haiti. Similar to the studies by Dr. Collins and Dr. David, Andrasfay and Goldman found that the babies of foreign-born Black women were heavier than US-born Black women with an average weight of 3,199 grams compared to 3,083 grams. The difference in the rates of low-birthweight babies between Black US-born and Black foreign-born mothers was 11.8% and 7.8%, respectively. When it came to the next generation, the grandchildren of the foreign-born Black women, the average birthweight was 3,032 grams compared to 3,020 grams for the grandchildren of US-born Black women. The differences in the rates of low-birthweight babies shrunk, with the rates being 12.2% and 13.1% for the two groups, respectively. While there was a decrease in the average birthweight for White and Hispanic women from G2 to G3, foreign-born Hispanic women saw a substantially smaller decline in birthweights compared to foreign-born Black women, and the narrowing of the gaps in the rates of low birthweight was markedly lower. The comparable rates of LBW between US-born and foreign-born Hispanic women were 6.2% and 4.5% for G2 babies, and 7.2% and 6.1% for G3 babies. For foreign-born White women, the rate of LBW for G3 was 6.1%; for G2 it was 5.3% compared to a G3 rate of 5.9% and 5.2% for US-born White women. The increased percentages of low birthweights for the G3 births among foreign-born Black women were particularly evident for less educated mothers, with progressively decreasing but substantial disparities noted for those whose highest completed level of education was less than high school, high school, and some college. Interestingly, the G2 births of foreign-born college-educated Black women had higher rates of LBW compared to their less educated peers; and although college education provided some protection for G3 births, compared to similarly educated mothers of G2 babies, the prevalence of low birthweights was only slightly better, at approximately 9.4% for college-educated mothers of G3 babies, compared to 10% for college-educated mothers of G2 babies and still higher than rates for the less educated Black foreign-born G2 mothers. Studies have shown that while foreign-born Black pregnant women face less discrimination than US-born Black pregnant women,[12] their children face the same levels of discrimination as their counterparts with US-born parents.[13] Furthermore, for a foreign-born pregnant woman who migrated to the United States before age eighteen, or was from the Caribbean, the self-reported racism was closer to that of their US-born counterparts.[14] It doesn't take long for racism in America to affect Black women, no matter where they are from.

Obviously, there is an overlap between low birthweight births and preterm births. Preterm babies often weigh less than 2,500 grams, depending on how many weeks before the full term they are born. It is estimated that two-thirds of low birthweight babies are premature.[15] On the other hand, a large percentage (almost 60%) of preterm babies are not low birthweight.[16] The other factor that affects the birthweight of babies is what happened to Linda Villarosa. Her baby did not grow as well as she should have inside the uterus, forcing her to be delivered preterm. Even if she were allowed to get to 37 weeks, her daughter would still be smaller than she should have been.

Historically, the rates of low birthweight babies had risen from 1990 to 2006 by almost 20%, but declined between 2007 and 2012. Since 2016, the rates have declined 2% for non-Hispanic (NH) White women but have increased 4% for NH Black women and 3% for Hispanic women.[17] The most recently reported CDC rates for 2020 were 6.84% for NH White women, 7.40% for Hispanic women, and 14.19% for Black women. It is interesting how the timing of the increase of LBW for Black and Hispanic women correlated with significant political changes in the country. I am hard-pressed to think that this is a mere coincidence.

Regardless of educational level, Black women in America have higher rates of LBW than any other racial/ethnic group no matter the educational level of that group, including NH American Indian and Alaska Native, NH Asian, NH Black, NH White, and Hispanic.[18]

In early 2017, I listened to a TED talk by Miriam Zoila Pérez. The talk, entitled the "How Racism Harms Pregnant Women—and What Can Help,"[19] was probably one of the most impactful TED talks I have ever listened to. It finally explained the infant-mortality health disparity that I noticed when I sat in the auditorium in medical school in the 1990s. For me, it was an Oprah-sized "aha" moment. Ms. Perez discussed the negative effect of racism on Black women and their babies. She offered a solution, "The JJ Way®." It was an innovation by Jennie Joseph, a British-trained midwife who migrated to the United States in 1989. Joseph implemented this model of care in her clinic in Orlando, Florida. The Health Council of East Central Florida evaluated the JJ Way® from 2006 to 2007. Of the one hundred patients who enrolled in the study, twenty-nine were African American. What was remarkable is that in this initial cohort no women who identified as African American or Black had a low birthweight baby or delivered preterm. However, the numbers of Black participants were small and that zero rate in both metrics occurred for seventeen Hispanic women as well. For the forty-six White women the rate was 4.8% and 4.7%, respectively. In a larger cohort of 256 patients who had care between February 2016 and 2017, 54.7% of whom were White and 36.3% were

Black or African American, the rate of low birthweight babies for Black women was 8.6%, compared to the rate of 13.1% in Orange County, Florida where the Jennie's clinic is located. The preterm birthrate among the same population of Black women was 8.6%, compared to 13% in Orange County. For White women, the rate of low birthweight was 2.8% compared to the 7.1% Orange County rate and for preterm birth it was 5% compared to 9%. The data was compiled by an independent consulting firm.[20] The JJ Way® has "four cornerstones: access, connection, knowledge, and empowerment."[21] The report detailed that no patient is denied care, regardless of their resources. Efforts are made to ensure that strong connections are forged between all the members of the care team, whether clinical or nonclinical, and the patients. Additionally, the participation of the father and the extended family and friend group of the patients is encouraged. Culturally sensitive education is provided in a variety of methods to improve knowledge, including providing group-based education in the waiting rooms. It is thought that the three cornerstones lead to patients' empowerment.

In the early 2000s, a program called Healthy Families New York was initiated to improve health outcomes for disadvantaged women and adolescents. Using that opportunity, researchers decided to perform a randomized control trial to evaluate the effect of home visitation on low birthweight.[22] Their research was informed by two earlier effective trials. The target population consisted of pregnant women and adolescents, many young, many unmarried, many first-time mothers who lived in disadvantaged communities with high rates of LBW babies among other risk factors. To be involved in this study, participants had to be enrolled in the larger program by week 30. Forty-one and a half percent of the women were Black, 24.6% were Hispanic, and 31.4% were White. The intervention group received home visits, and the control group was "given information and referrals to services other than home visitation."[23] The home visits were biweekly and lasted for approximately one hour. The visitors were trained for the role and often had experience with babies and young children, but they were not healthcare professionals. Only half had some college education. The visits focused on three activities: improving the "mother's social support, providing prenatal education, and linking the mother to other services in the community."[24] The visitors helped mothers establish trusted social networks; decrease stress; promote healthy habits, including healthy nutrition and avoiding risky behaviors such as drug use, smoking, and drinking; helped to make sure the mothers had access to the consistent prenatal care they needed and that they attended those visits. In addition, the visitors linked the mothers to other tangible support such as food stamps and the Special Supplemental Nutrition Program for Women, Infants, and Children (WIC). The rate of LBW was 5.1% in the intervention group versus 9.8% in the control group. If the women were randomized before 16 weeks, and as such received the intervention longer and more home visits, the rates of LBW were 3.6% in the intervention group versus 14.1% in the control group. Of the three racial/ethnic groups of mothers examined, the intervention was most effective for Black mothers. Their LBW rates were 3.1% in the intervention group versus 10.2% in the control group. The rate of reduction of LBW in the other groups studied, while trending lower, did not reach statistical significance.

I mentioned two earlier trials which informed the researchers in the New York study. One of the studies was published in 1996. LBW is not a new problem in the Black community. They specifically targeted low-income African American women in Alameda County, California, who were determined to be at risk of having "inadequate social support."[25] The included women were all low-income, determined by eligibility for Medicaid; they were between 16 and 26 weeks of pregnancy and were ages eighteen to thirty-four. The only health problem the study excluded was "major mental illness."[26] They included women with singleton pregnancies and excluded them if their pregnancies ended before 20 weeks, whether voluntarily or via miscarriage. They found 114 women who met their criteria. About half received the intervention, which consisted of four face-to-face sessions provided by registered nurses which occurred approximately every 2 weeks and telephone calls in between. The control group had standard prenatal care and did not know what the intervention involved. The sessions focused on different aspects of the pregnant women's social support. "The first session was an interview that provided assessment and validation of the woman's life situation and social supports by focusing on three problem areas and three successful areas in the woman's life, along with an exploration of the social supports associated with each of these areas."[27] Other sessions focused on issues such self-esteem and types of relationships. The rate of LBW was 9.1% in the intervention group and 22.4% in the control group, as compared to the Alameda County rates of 14% for African Americans and 5% for Caucasians within the same period.

The study authors suggested that when offering social support, it is important to identify women who need it. This needs assessment can be completed with preexisting criteria sets. The authors also emphasized the need to recognize cultural differences in selecting effective support persons.

The third trial involved a two-year follow-up to evaluate the efficacy of support by paraprofessionals, as compared to nurses, for low-income pregnant women in Denver, Colorado, in the 1990s.[28] All the pregnant women were new to motherhood and were Medicaid-eligible. Approximately 47% of the women were Mexican American, 15% were Black, 35% were White, and 3% were American/Indian/Asian. Eighty-five percent of the women were unmarried. The paraprofessionals needed to have a high school education, "no college preparation in helping professions" and strong "people skills." There were two supervisors for every ten paraprofessionals. The paraprofessionals visited the women approximately six times during the pregnancy and sixteen visits during the first two years of the child's life. The nurses visited the mothers on average six and a half times during the pregnancy and twenty-one times during the first two years of the child's life. While the women who were visited by the nurse reported less domestic violence from their partners and slightly longer interval between children—24.5 months versus 20.4 months without any intervention—there were multiple noteworthy findings for the women visited by paraprofessionals. If the women got pregnant again, they were less likely to miscarry or have a low birthweight baby. They also reported better mental health, despite having lower rates of marriage and cohabitation with the child's father. Interestingly, the authors appeared to discount the benefits of the paraprofessionals and did not recommend an investment in paraprofessionals.

Technically, my children are G3 births. My risk of low birthweight could have approached 15% when I consider the rates of Black women in America in my age group in the years my children were born. My risk may have lowered because of my education, since that at least helped the daughters of foreign-born Black women. When I think about my adult life leading up to the birth of my children, I had a mixture of mitigating and aggravating factors: factors that could have worsened my pregnancy-related risk and risk of low birthweight and factors that I am sure now were protective, but there was one mitigating factor I valued above all others.

My obstetrics and gynecology residency was one of the most stressful periods of my professional life. It was stressful because of overt personal attacks and microaggressions that I later realized were due to my presence as a Black female Ivy League graduate. However, the stress was also largely due to the demands of the work, which involved doing all-night shifts that extended to 5 p.m. the following day, as often as every other night, in addition to learning the specialty and the need to perform well. My buffer was my social circle. In the Washington DC, Maryland, and Virginia (DMV) area, I was able to find multiple like-minded friends. Socializing together was a big priority. My friend network made almost unbearable moments bearable. My friends helped to silence the early thoughts I had of leaving my program. Though my first job out of residency was technically easier, I left after two years because I noticed the relative dearth of social support was adversely affecting my state of mind and well-being. I returned to my safe haven, the DMV area. I was not disappointed. Again, my social network buffered against life stressors.

I had spent more than ten years in the United States before I returned to Jamaica. Despite the support of my family, there were challenges. My only professional choice was to start my own solo OB/GYN practice. My social network had narrowed considerably over the years. Gradually, I regrew my network, mainly through my membership in a service club, the Rotary Club of Kingston. Service to others had provided an almost unquantifiable service to me. I found a large social network by attending the weekly luncheon meetings. As we worked to support the less economically advantaged, we fellowshipped with one another. It was friends from that same network who introduced me to my husband. This was the same network that I had when I carried both my children. They supplemented the support of my family, a few longtime close friends and a very supportive husband.

Why do I make this point in relationship to low birthweight babies? A common thread of successful interventions I described is social support. Jennie Joseph created a center that not only provided prenatal care but was a hub of social support. The successful New York intervention involved home visitation from community members, none of whom were healthcare professionals. The California intervention was formulated from an observation of limited success of medical interventions to improve LBW and deliberated used models from the social support literature. The Denver intervention improved LBW only with visits by paraprofessionals and not nurses.

In the two years between the time I got married and gave birth to my first child, my social network was the area of my life that I felt most comfortable about. I still had the stress of growing a solo OB/GYN practice and writing a regular health column for a major newspaper. I tried to eat a version of a healthy diet, but nothing close to the diet I have learned about in the past few years, and I exercised intermittently. Being in Jamaica during that time, I do not recall any experiences of racial discrimination. My buffers were more than able to compensate for my stressors. Based on what I know now, I believe it was integral to me having almost perfect birth outcomes despite age-related and even occupational risks.[29]

Black women in America cannot usually escape the racial discrimination of this country to protect their pregnancies by moving to another country like I was able to do. They cannot escape the racism that can potentially cripple their children's life course from even before they emerge to meet this world. My daughter is an American kid. Jamaica is not home to her like it was to me. How can I support her if she decides to have children when she grows up? How can I help to ensure that she, as a Black woman in America, can have a normal-birthweight baby? The same way that I suggest we support pregnant Black women in America.

Of course, we should ensure that pregnant Black women have access to unbiased prenatal care; of course, we should ensure that they are provided with culturally sensitive prenatal education; of course, we should close the gap on access to resources, such as healthy food and housing (we should have been doing that already), *and* we should strengthen the social support. We should provide funding for community home visitations during pregnancy to the most vulnerable mothers. Based on the available research, there is good evidence that low-income Black women would gain the most support from trained individuals from within their own community or from similar communities. A college education is not required for these community workers. It offers post-high-school opportunities even to individuals who plan to move on to college at a later time. We should establish more prenatal-care centers employing key elements of the JJ Way®, or implement these elements in existing prenatal-care settings with similar demographics, such as federally qualified health centers. Professional Black women are in no less need of support. We should establish easily accessible social networks for pregnant Black professional women with choices for women to find their niche, a group they feel comfortable with. These networks can be patterned off the multiple existing networks that Black women engage with currently.

Do Black women in America need this additional support more than other racial groups? They do! A Black woman in America needs as many buffers as possible. If she is economically disadvantaged, she may face stressors related to food and housing security, neighborhood safety, and overt and implicit biases in multiple settings, including at her prenatal visit. Economically advantaged Black women face the constant pressure of having to outperform their non-Black peers to get the same, or even lower, levels of recognition, and despite their professional accomplishments they may be exposed to the same explicit and implicit biases when they seek healthcare. Can buffers be provided by the healthcare system and auxiliary support systems? Jennie Josephs and others have shown us that the answer is again, yes, they can.

CHAPTER 10

Social Support for Black Pregnant Women and the Role of the Father

Growing up, I had clear goals for my future. As you already know, my first desire to be a doctor came at age seven, and I was absolutely certain of my calling by age thirteen. I was equally certain that I wanted to be married. Perhaps like many Catholic girls going to Catholic schools at that time, I briefly entertained the thought of entering the convent. Maybe it's more appropriate to say, fleetingly. I was sold on the story of Cinderella in my early childhood years, and I wanted to meet my knight in shining armor—even if my Cinderella story would involve me being a doctor rather than running a palace. If I could use one word to describe my journey to meeting my husband Ryan, it would be "rough." So rough that it inspired me to write my second book, *Please God Send Me a Husband,* to help other women.

I struggled as a Black woman to find someone I considered a suitable partner. I wanted someone who valued tertiary education in the way I did, shared my faith, and, given my Catholic background, I was more comfortable if he was not divorced. His race and ethnicity did not matter—at least I did not think they were significant. Looking back, I realized I added unnecessary criteria. I remember, early in my professional career I was at a club in Washington, DC, with some friends. I ran into some medical students whom I had taught. They attended the Walter Reed Medical Center, now called the F. Edward Herbert School of Medicine. The teaching relationship had long ended, and they were at an institution that was separate from my own. One of the students approached me and informed me that his friend, another student, had a crush on me. He was a handsome White male with an engaging personality, and he was an excellent student. I had no idea of his interest in me during the rotation, and he was always appropriate during our interactions. I felt flattered, but in seeking to uphold an ethical standard I did not bother to explore or ask questions. Another friend asked me to dance, and I chose to accept. I meant to get back to that student, but they had left. I intended to get back to him, not because of the rules I felt I had to follow, but rather to ensure that I let him know I appreciated his willingness to share his interest in me.

Contrary to my own reluctance to date a former student, I recall a White colleague in residency ultimately marrying someone who had been a medical student from the same program. While I am sure she observed all the necessary protocols, clearly, she did not dismiss the student's interest as quickly as I had dismissed this other young man. While I recognize that I had placed some of my own constraints, given the position of that young man as a former student, I can't help but wonder if my reluctance to be open to him was further fueled by concern about the extra scrutiny I would receive as a Black professional woman in America.

Yet, I was lucky. I met and married a man who has been an exceptional life partner and a supportive husband and father to our two children. Since I was already in my mid-thirties when we met, we candidly discussed our openness to adoption, should we be unsuccessful in our attempts to have children biologically.

Many Black women I know, patients, friends, and acquaintances, were not so lucky. They did not meet the "right man" in time. For some, relationships that showed promise ended prematurely, and for others, the life partner they hoped for never came along. For some, the pregnancy may not have been planned, but they chose to continue their pregnancy despite the almost certain knowledge that the father would never be a part of their lives; while others took matters in their own hands and used reproductive technologies to ensure they gave birth to children before biology failed them—without the promise of a life partner in sight.

Do Black women have more difficulty finding marital partners than other women? They do! To be clear, I am not referring to women who make the deliberate choice to remain unpartnered or women who choose same-sex relationships. I am referring to those who desired a husband, but felt they had to make the best of a situation that fell far short of their ideals.

It's disappointing how the United States has systematically set Black women up to be single parents, while at the same time imposing a negative stereotype on Black women who are single parents.

Going back to slavery, it was not legal for enslaved people to get married; however, they found other ways to formalize their unions. In northern states, African Americans could marry after slavery ended in 1830; but most African Americans lived in the south and could not legally marry until 1865 and later when slavery had ended in the rest of the country. Families lived under the constant threat of being separated; children could be snatched away from their parents completely or left with only a mother or a father. Even if the parents were present, they had to spend long hours on the plantation, forced to entrust the care of their children to others.[1] I can't help but wonder how that legacy has affected the descendants of enslaved people through this day.

Over the years, African American children have always been more likely than White children to live in a single-parent home, primarily with their mothers. Between 1880 and 1940, 13 to 14% of Black children between the ages of 0 and 14 were living with their mothers, compared to only 5 to 6% of White children. In 1960, the percentage was 18.2%, compared to 5.9%; and in 1980, this number had risen to 37.3% compared to 11.7%.[2] It is noteworthy that this data did not identify why a mother might be on her own; for example, in the 1960s, Black men were more likely to be drafted to the Vietnam War than White men and, at least in 1965, they were more likely to die.[3] Not to mention the many other ways Black men were targeted on American soil—targeting that still happens today, though fortunately to a lesser extent. Were some of the increased percentages of Black children living only with their mother between 1940 and 1960 due to the fact that Black women had lost their husbands to death? Years which marked the increase of Black children in single parent homes also showed a decrease in the percentage of Black families living in extended households, from 25.4% in 1960 to 17.2% in 1980. Extended households can include living with parents, siblings, or in-laws. I think it is most tragic that as the number of Black women who face pregnancy and parenting alone has increased, that extended family support appeared to decrease as well.

Based on 2020 Census Bureau data, 46.3% of Black children live with their mother only compared to 13.4% of White children.[4] Only 37.9% of Black children live with married parents, compared with 75.5% of White children. Of note, the percentage of children who live with White or Black parents who live together (unmarried) is about the same, 3.1% for White children and 3.4% for Black children.

Why do many Black women face parenting alone, and why has that trend been increasing over the years? Is it that they do not want to get married?

Sociologists have offered interesting statistics and explanations. Research suggests that more Black mothers perceive marriage to be beneficial than White mothers. However, Black mothers are less optimistic of their chances of being married.[5] Their lack of optimism can be supported by actual statistics. Black women are less likely to get married than other racial and ethnic groups including White, Asian, American Indian/ Native Alaskan, and Hispanic women whether US- or foreign-born.[6] The average age of marriage is four years older for Black women than for White women, thirty versus twenty-six. At ages forty to forty-four, years which may mark the last, often difficult, chance to give birth to a biological child, 34% of Black women have never been married, compared to 7% of White women. Black women are also more likely to have their marriages end in divorce than White women. The lower marriage rates for Black women have been partially explained by a few factors. One factor is imprisonment: Black men were more than five times as likely to be incarcerated as White men in 2018, despite a substantial drop in their incarceration rate since 2006.[7] Another is partner choice.

Americans are more likely to marry someone of their own race. However, while a larger percentage of Black people in America are more likely to marry outside their race (18% in 2015 versus 5% in 1980), Black men are twice as likely as Black women to have a spouse of a different race or ethnicity (24% versus 12%). Furthermore, both White and Hispanic men are equally likely as White and Hispanic women to marry outside their race, with Asian men being almost half as likely to marry outside their race as Asian women.[8] All of which further diminishes the potential pool of spouses for Black women.

An additional factor relates to education. Women tend to seek partners with similar education. I have already mentioned that this was a criterion I valued highly. Both White and Black women tend to be more educated than White and Black men, respectively; however, not only is the disparity in educational status greater for Black women than for White women,[9] but Black men with a college degree or higher are even more likely to marry interracially. In 2015, 30% of Black men with a bachelor's degree or higher married interracially, compared to 13% of Black women with the equivalent education.[10]

This still does not tell the entire story. Due to the higher mortality rates of Black men, there are fewer Black men between the ages of twenty-five and fifty-four, approximately 15% less, than there are Black women,[11] even though a more even distribution between males and females exists at younger ages. Furthermore, Black men are less likely to get married than their White and Hispanic counterparts, even if they are highly educated;[12] although their likelihood of getting married increases with their educational status. In 2012, only 57.6% of Black men between the ages of forty and forty-four, with less than twelve years of education, were married, compared to 77.6% of similarly educated White men. For Black men and White men with sixteen or more years of education, the difference was 76.5% and 85.5%, respectively.

I know a number of Black men who fall into that last statistic. I asked one of my friends who chose to be open with me. He is over the age of forty-five and has never been married, although he remains interested. He had a strong example of a successful marriage in his parents, who were married for many years before they passed away. He acknowledges that maybe he had "too many expectations" and the bar was set too high. Again, I wonder how his experience as a Black man in America contributed to those expectations and him setting such a high bar.

I must confess I agree with Stanford Law Professor Richard Banks who discussed in a paper why he thought interracial marriage is good for Black women.[13] He also suggested that some Black men are less likely to marry due to the multitude of dating options they have available. If a Black man ends a relationship, he has many options to start a new one.

But why do I feel the need to highlight the disparity in the rates of Black women being unmarried? The frank answer is because it can have a negative impact on their pregnancies.

In 1990, researchers published a study examining how being unmarried affected birth outcomes specifically for Black women.[14] Having already been aware that unmarried mothers had more adverse outcomes, they wanted to decipher whether those unmarried women simply tended to have more of other risk factors, or whether being unmarried was a risk factor in itself. They examined the births of over 36,608 mothers which occurred in Washington, DC, from 1980 to 1984. In their sample, 59% of the women were unmarried. While they noticed that married women were more likely to be older, have at least some college education, and benefit from adequate prenatal care, despite controlling for these variables, unmarried women were still more likely to give birth to low birthweight babies compared to married women. A meta-analysis published more recently, in 2010, showed that unmarried women were more likely to have an increased risk of low birthweight, preterm birth, and small-for-gestational-age births than married women, even when the unmarried woman lived with the biologic father of their child.[15] Being unmarried can even affect maternal mortality rates, with unmarried women in America having almost twice the maternal mortality rates as married women,[16] although the impact appears to be lesser for Black women possibly because of the myriad of other factors leading to their already disparately high rates.

While I do not expect that this particular social inequity that Black women face can be repaired in the short term, what can we do now to mitigate the negative effects of Black women facing pregnancy alone?

A few years ago, I read a powerful, well-researched essay written by Linda Villarosa. It was published in the *New York Times Magazine* under the title "Why America's Black Mothers and Babies are in a Life-or-Death Crisis."[17] It described the story of Simone Landrum, a young single mother in New Orleans, with a difficult childhood and an abusive relationship, who lost her baby, Harmony, due to placental abruption (a complication that involves the separation of the placenta from the wall of the uterus). Based on the story, the placental abruption appeared to be due to high blood pressure associated with the pregnancy complication, preeclampsia (discussed in chapter 7) not being diagnosed in a timely manner. After her loss, she was able to flee the abusive relationship but got pregnant the following year in a new, but short-lived, relationship. She was paired with a doula due to the thoughtful intervention of her case manager. Her doula, Latona Giwa, provided support to her during the last one to two months of her pregnancy, her labor and delivery, and made six postpartum visits. Latona Giwa was particularly experienced in childbirth having worked as a labor and delivery nurse. Ms. Giwa provided unparalleled support including advocacy and support in the hospital and even addressing social needs such as taking Ms. Landrum home after her full-term vaginal delivery, supplying her with immediate food and groceries, ensuring that Ms. Landrum had scheduled her postpartum visit, and even discussing contraception.

Before reading that article, I had merely thought of doulas as a luxury that more affluent White women afforded themselves to allow them to have a more "natural" childbirth experience with lower medical interventions. I had concerns that doulas would overly interfere with patient care leading to more difficult patient–doctor interactions without benefiting the patient. Linda Villarosa's article was illuminating. Research including some cited by Villarosa and others not only confirms that doulas can decrease cesarean section rates,[18] which I will touch on in chapter 14, but can reduce preterm birth.[19]

Other studies have demonstrated that doula-assisted mothers are four times less likely to have a low birthweight baby and more likely to initiate breastfeeding in a group of mothers who primarily identified as African American.[20] In this study, all mothers were offered doulas, and the comparisons were made between the mothers who chose to have doulas versus those who did not. The doulas sometimes attended childbirth education classes with the mothers, but all doulas met with the mothers twice before birth, offered continuous assistance throughout labor and birth, and visited them at least two times postpartum. The doula-supported mothers were slightly older, with an average age of 20.3 versus 19.1 for non-doula mothers. Non-doula mothers were more likely to be living with their family or guardian, compared to doula mothers who were more likely to be living with partners or nonfamily. Interestingly, although doula mothers expected more support from someone close to them, in comparison to non-doula mothers, they still wanted the additional support of a doula. Additionally, doula support showed promise in decreasing birth complications involving the mother or baby, although the study did not specifically identify which complications. Like all research studies, this study has limitations, including the fact there may be other unidentified differences between women who chose doulas versus those who did not. Nonetheless, the results are encouraging.

But is doula support available to women? For many, the answer is: not nearly enough. However, there is reason to be optimistic, since with continued advocacy at least some states, including Florida, Maryland, Minnesota, New Jersey, and Oregon,[21] cover doula services for pregnant women with Medicaid. Many other states are implementing coverage or have taken legislative action. Employer-based health plans appear to be further behind. Employers need to consider the disparate adverse health risks that Black women face and ensure that they provide the option of doula support for their employees. The extent of the subsidy could be tied to need or risk factors through the equity lens. It really is so much cheaper to cover the cost of a doula than to cover the cost of the complications that they may help to prevent.

Since moving to Connecticut, I had the pleasure to connect with SciHonor Devotion, a doula and educator. She established Earth's Natural Touch: Birth Care and Beyond, a doula collective that operates in thirteen states.[22] Through her advocacy, and those of others, she has managed to obtain some funding from the March of Dimes and New Haven Healthy Start (a federally funded initiative which "focuses on infant mortality and eliminating racial and ethnic disparities in birth outcome"[23]) to provide families with some support; but providing doula services to mothers who are unable to afford it has been challenging.

Of course, doula support is not the only form of intervention that can improve some of the outcomes that Black unmarried women face, such as preterm deliveries or low birthweight babies (as I have already discussed in chapters 5 and 9) but what else can be done to support single Black pregnant women?

In chapter 8 on stillbirth, I mentioned the benefits of community health committees to decrease stillbirth rates. This is not the only benefit. "Community based intervention packages involving family members through community support and advocacy groups and community mobilization along with additional training of outreach workers was reported as one of the most successful strategies showing significant impacts on maternal morbidity"[24] (negative health consequences that mothers suffer due to pregnancy related issues). What can that support look like? Based on the research, I think it is important to start the work within existing frameworks: family and friend networks, community centers, or churches. Next, volunteers can be recruited for pregnancy-support committees or, if those committees already exist, evaluate their strengths and build on areas for improvement. Volunteers should have enhanced education on pregnancy warning signs so that they not only can encourage pregnant women to get help in a timely manner but improve the understanding of what specific symptoms could mean. Committees could support families with healthy meals, childcare assistance, and/or ideally home visits to provide a sometimes-overlooked social outlet for expectant mothers. Successful interventions should be documented and built on.

I discussed extensively support that can be used to supplement the role of absent fathers, but how can the many fathers, who remain present, be supported? What do they need to know?

Dr. Sally Ward, whose postpartum story I will describe in chapter 15 cited at least three occasions where her husband's support and encouragement, at the minimum, led her to seek medical help, which may have saved her life. While I may not be able to quantify in absolute terms how my husband's support helped me in my pregnancies, I know he was a sounding board, a buffer for stress throughout my pregnancies, and a constant bedside companion throughout my hospital stays.

The partners of Black pregnant women need to be acknowledged and their importance endorsed. Whenever possible, they should be encouraged to participate in prenatal appointments, even if these appointments are remote. Healthcare professionals, with patients' consent, need to address the concerns of the partners as well. Educational pregnancy programs should be designed to specifically address partners' unique needs and concerns.

Years ago, I had the pleasure to hear from the father of quadruplets (four babies born at the same time). He detailed how the bonding with his children began when he heard his babies' heartbeats for the first time. I fondly remember the many years of my private practice when many of my patients attended prenatal visits with their spouses. I felt I was not just getting to know a mother, my patient, but a family. Workplaces need to allow spouses the opportunity to support their pregnant partners, not just in the delivery but throughout the pregnancy and postpartum. Paternity leave needs to be expanded for fathers without ignoring those in low-income positions. When the partners of Black pregnant women are ready and willing to step into their role, they should not be sabotaged—especially when we know the important role they play in the protecting the health of their partners and their future children.

Bethany Stone* had her whole future ahead of her, and it looked bright. She was twenty-three years old, had finished college just over a year before, but had stayed in the same town, waiting tables at a popular restaurant while she saved for business school. The local bar was a popular after-work hangout spot for her and her friends. Jake seldom hung out there, but he knew many of her friends from high school. He was an attractive guy, six years older and in graduate school. They dated for a few months and became sexually intimate. Right after, they both knew it was a mistake, it was too soon. But for Bethany it was already too late, she was pregnant. They had sex only once. She told Jake about the pregnancy, but he panicked. He didn't want her to keep the child. Her mind was made up. She was having the baby with or without him.

"Is it my race?," she candidly asked. Jake was White and Bethany was Black. He adamantly denied that race was an issue; but it didn't matter, he was not going to be involved. Bethany scrambled to get insurance. The restaurant where she worked provided subsidies for insurance, but she was young and healthy, she hadn't thought she was going to need it. She was wrong. Fortunately, she lived in a state that had good Medicaid benefits, and she was able to get her appropriate tests and prenatal visits. She shared the news with her family—all of whom lived out of state—when she saw them on a holiday visit. If her parents were disappointed, they did not let her know it. They jumped to her aid, offering encouragement that this was not going to derail her life goals. She would still go to the business school. Nevertheless, with a strong traditional Christian background, it is unlikely this is what they envisioned for their little girl.

Bethany realized that going home to her parents was not the best option. It was a small town with limited opportunities for a pregnant woman. She intended to do it alone. Her sister-in-law was not having it. Having recently given birth to her first child, she knew pregnancy, and new motherhood was not an easy journey. She insisted that Bethany live with her and her husband, Bethany's brother, who was more than willing to help to support his baby sister.

Bethany packed up and moved to their state by her 17th week of pregnancy. Jobless, she again needed to seek state insurance, but fortunately she qualified. She soon found employment, and with her room and board covered by her brother and his wife, she was able to save for the baby. She found an obstetrician and was able to continue her care with him for the remainder of the pregnancy. She liked her doctor, a White male, and had no complaints about his care.

Her pregnancy went well. Despite the father not being involved, she had the support of her family and friends. The healthcare team noticed placenta previa (a condition where the placenta covers the opening of the uterus) early in the pregnancy, but it resolved well before the delivery. She caught chicken pox from someone at work. Fortunately, with about 8 weeks to go till her delivery, it didn't cause any harm to her developing baby, and she made an excellent recovery.

Two days before her due date she started to experience cramps. Her brother and sister were out, but she was in the capable hands of her friend Amber, who was visiting from law school. She went to the hospital about four hours later. It was about midnight. She was only dilated two centimeters and after observing her for several hours without change they sent her home at about 6 a.m. They insisted that she should not return until the contractions were two minutes apart. She continued to labor that day, not eating and barely drinking, she had no appetite for food. Twenty-four hours had gone by since her labor had started, but the contractions still were not two minutes apart. Her sister-in-law intervened:

"This is ridiculous, I'm taking you back."

She was in pain, but her cervical exam had changed little. Nevertheless, she was admitted. As the pain intensified, she was ready for an epidural. She remembers being told that she could not get it because she had Medicaid. Consumed with pain, she had no strength to fight. But she didn't have to. Amber stepped in. Fresh out of law school, she employed all her newly minted legal skills.

"This person is in pain, and you need to do whatever you need to do to make it better!" Soon after, the anesthesiologist came in. A few hours later, Bethany was ready. She remembers waiting for her doctor crossed-legged because she was sure the baby would come out. Her primary obstetrician was on vacation, but his female partner came in for the delivery. She delivered by the third push. Her doctor remarked as soon as her baby was born: "Where did you get that baby with those blond eyebrows?"

"I guess she thought because I was a Black woman it had to be a Black baby," Bethany remarked in retelling her story. Bethany's family and friends continued to rally around her during her postpartum course, and she only had venture to live on her own again with her young baby when she was ready. Bethany did complete business school and earned additional graduate degrees since then. As for her baby, that child grew up and went on to graduate from a prestigious university.

Women often have to face pregnancy alone, Black women even more so. It is not that they have to be married or have the father present to get optimal social support. If single women, or women in same-sex relationships, choose to parent, their support can come from other relationships, whether these relationships are marital, intimate, or platonic. Bethany felt cared for by her brother and his wife because they opened their home to her; provided her with meals and lodging; allowed her to allocate her savings to future care for her baby; remained mindful of her needs as a young soon-to-be mother, support which continued in the postpartum period. Support can come from other family members or friends. It can come from the community. It can come from religious organizations. If we, as a society, invested our energy and resources into supporting Black pregnant women, rather than judging them, I'm certain that collectively we would be much better off.

CHAPTER 11

Sickle Cell Disease and Lupus— Ignored and Undertreated

Connie* had been a patient of mine for a few years while I was practicing in Jamaica. She was young and full of promise. She came into
my office to announce to me that she was pregnant. She was no longer
going to be in my care because she knew her pregnancy would be high
risk due to her sickle cell disease (SCD), and she was going to continue
her pregnancy care at the university hospital. She had a type called
hemoglobin SCD. It is usually a less severe form of SCD. I called my
colleague who was a specialist in maternal fetal medicine, high-risk
obstetrics. I knew I had placed my patient in capable hands. However,
several months later, I got a terrible call from my colleague. Connie had
died. She had given birth to a healthy infant, but within days of delivery
she developed pneumonia and succumbed to the disease. The image of
Connie telling me she was pregnant reverberates in my mind. I often
wonder if Connie would have lived if she had received care from some
of the state-of-the-art tertiary institutions where I had worked in the
United States. But I am not so sure.

Sickle cell disease "is a group of inherited red blood cell disorders.
In SCD, the red blood cells become hard and sticky and look like a
C-shaped farm tool called a 'sickle.'"[1] These abnormal cells die more
quickly than healthy red blood cells, leading to anemia. Their abnormal
shape can lead to blockage of the blood flow through blood vessels,
which can lead to other serious complications. SCD predominantly
affects people of African descent. If most of the patients who have a
specific condition are of a certain race or ethnicity, I think it stands

to reason that most of the experience acquired or therapies developed would have resulted from treating that race and condition. I think of a condition like cystic fibrosis, a very serious lung condition, most common in White patients. In the 1960s the average life expectancy was as low as fifteen, it moved to thirty-one in the 1990s, and now it is forty-six years.[2] The same was true for sickle cell disease, at least at first. Lanzrkon et al. published a study in 2013 where they evaluated whether there had been improvements in survival for adults who had sickle cell disease over the years from 1979 to 2005.[3] They shared that in the 1970s, the average life expectancy was less than twenty. In the 1990s, it increased to a median age of forty-eight for women. Since then, the authors noted that an effective treatment had been available to treat sickle cell disease. The authors specifically wanted to evaluate how the mortality rates had changed since the development of that medication.[4] They got worse. In 2005, the median life expectancy for women decreased to forty-two. Even more disturbing was the fact that the adult mortality rate was higher than it was in 1979.

My friend Claudia Ferguson was a strong advocate for the disease. She lived in Florida. In March 2021 she posted: "I was hospitalized two weeks ago and I'm literally having nightmares regarding my stay.... I personally thought that things were improving. So this has been like a shock to me."[5] She highlighted the stigma which people with the disease faced and the lack of compassion of healthcare professionals. People with the condition have intense pain crisis. The stigma includes them being labeled as drug seekers.[6] Within days of that post, Claudia died. She was forty-eight years old.

Claudia never dared to have children. She never dared to place what she considered the burden of her illness on a spouse, so she remained unpartnered despite having loved and having been loved.

Would her care have been better if she had become pregnant? Is the care any better for pregnant Black women with sickle cell disease? Again, the answer is, it is not. A cross-sectional analysis was performed to assess severe maternal morbidity (SMM) for Black versus non-Black patients.[7] The rate of SMM for patients with sickle cell anemia already far exceeded the rate for those without the disease, with a rate of 45.58% for those with the disease compared to 1.49% for those without the disease, and for every year studied, 2007 to 2013, it was worse for Black people than for non-Black people. Black women faced risk of severe maternal morbidity twice as high as non-Black women did. It seems that if you have a "Black" disease in America you fall to the back of the line, but you are in double jeopardy if you are a Black person with a "Black" disease.

Lupus (systemic lupus erythematosus) is not necessarily a "Black" disease, but it is most prevalent in Black women. Estimates from the early 2000s place it as six times more common in women versus men, with African American women twice as likely to have it as White women.[8] I don't recall caring for many pregnant women with this disease throughout my career. Usually, they would be cared for by high-risk obstetricians. The person I recall who suffered from the disease was a classmate from school. I don't know what age she developed lupus, but I know she was young. I remember seeing her running an errand in a public office building. She was in her early thirties. We had a brief conversation, she told me she was tired. She meant tired from the demands of the debilitating illness she had. Within weeks of the time our paths had crossed she was dead. I remarked to her close friend: "She told me she was tired, maybe she was ready." Her friend said, "No, she was not ready, she wanted to live like everyone else." She too did not have the opportunity to have a family, to have children.

Lupus usually affects women in the years they would like to have a family, and many desire to have children. My former classmate may have, too. If she did, that dream died with her.

While lupus does not necessarily get worse in pregnancy, similar to women with SCD, women with lupus are more likely to have complications in pregnancy. For the years 2000 to 2003, a study showed that the risks included a greater than 36% cesarean section rate, a 22.5% preeclampsia rate, and a 20% rate of preterm labor[9]—complications which already occur more frequently in Black pregnant women. It should be no surprise that Black pregnant women with lupus have it worse than non-Black women.

A study evaluating the racial disparities in complications rate between 2008 and 2010 was published a few years later by Dr. Megan Clowse,[10] the same lead author of the earlier studies. Like she had done for her earlier publication, she used the Nationwide Inpatient Sample (NIS) for her data source. There were more White pregnant women than Black pregnant women in the sample, but lupus pregnancies accounted for a higher proportion of the pregnancies of Black women compared to the pregnancies of White women: 1.86 per 1,000 Black deliveries compared to 1.04 per 1,000 White deliveries. Over the years, some of the complications rates had changed. For example, the overall cesarean section rate had increased, much like it had for women with all levels of risk, something I will discuss further in chapter 14. It was more than 40%: 42% for Black women and 41.4% for White women. In this case, the rates for Hispanic women were even worse, at 47.6%.

Interestingly, preeclampsia rates were slightly better: less than 20%; but the racial disparity remained, with a rate of 13.5% for White women and 19% for Black women. The preterm labor rates were 24.7% for Black women and 14.3% for White women. Black babies were almost twice as likely to have poor growth in the uterus (fetal growth restriction). Coming into the pregnancy, Black women had higher rates of chronic hypertension and chronic renal failure, despite the fact that they were less likely to smoke, a behavior which can exacerbate their condition. This might suggest that before they became pregnant their lupus care had been suboptimal.

When I think of conditions like SCD and lupus, I think even more of the importance of advocacy and passion in making change in healthcare. There are many conditions that adversely affect the lives of Black pregnant women and women in general. Some conditions like hypertensive disorders are more common and invariably we hear more about them. While none of the conditions are getting the attention they need, I still don't want us to forget the less common ones: those that prematurely cut the lives of proportionately more Black women; those that deny them the chance of bearing their own children or, for those women who do try, make their risk of having a complication and dying greater than ever. Claudia Ferguson's advocacy made me think about more about SCD, a condition I rarely saw in clinical care.

Yvette Fay Francis-McBarnette was a Jamaican-born pioneer in the treatment of sickle cell disease. At only nineteen years old, she was the second Black woman to matriculate at Yale Medical School. Yet despite our shared commonalities, Jamaican-born parents and affiliation with Yale, I would have never known about her were it not for serendipity or fate. I interacted with Dr. Francis-McBarnette toward to tail-end of her life. In the capacity that I met her, I would not have known her history. One of her daughters, who was with her during the interaction, suggested that I read about her, which I promptly did. Dr. Francis-McBarnette pioneered the use of antibiotics to treat sickle cell anemia, became the director of the sickle cell anemia clinic at Jamaica Hospital in New York, and served on a White House advisory committee under President Nixon.[11] The work of the committee led to increased funding for education, screening, funding, and research on the condition. Dr. Francis-McBarnette originally trained as a pediatrician, but in order to continue to provide care to her patients into their adulthood, she went on to complete training in internal medicine and hematology starting at the age of fifty-two. The patients she cared for lived substantially longer than what was expected;[12] some had gone on to safely have children and enjoy educational success.[13] Physician advocates remain.

A few years before she died, Claudia felt that it was important that she connect me with Dr. Lanetta Bronté-Hall. She felt that Dr. Bronté-Hall was doing good work. Dr. Bronté-Hall grew up in a small town in North Carolina. She knew she wanted to be a scientist even before she went to college. In graduate school at the University of North Carolina, Chapel Hill, she studied parasites and was fascinated by the fact that people with sickle cell trait had protection again malaria. This realization generated her initial interest in the disease. Working with a mentor in graduate school, she had the opportunity to attend a medical clinic with him. While there, knowing her experience as a phlebotomist, her mentor tasked her with collecting blood from one of his patients. The patient was a young Black man, and working in predominantly White institutions, she was struck by the fact that the patient looked just like her. She now saw the connection between blood she had analyzed in the past and the human beings whom the blood belonged to.

Dr. Bronté-Hall went on to complete her degree in medical parasitology and laboratory practice. This was followed by a medical degree and a master's in public health. Despite completing her internship in internal medicine at Tulane University School of Medicine and residency in psychiatry at the University of Miami, Miller School of Medicine, she knew that she initially wanted to go into administration; nevertheless, her commitment to sickle cell disease remained. Currently she is the President and Chief Health Officer of the Foundation for Sickle Cell Disease Research.[14] Among other services, the foundation offers urgent care for management of acute pain crises. It also gives patients the opportunity to participate in research on the disease. She notes that her patients are eager participants. Between 2021 and 2022, working with high-risk obstetric specialists, she had the pleasure to participate in the care of three pregnant patients with sickle cell disease. All three had uncomplicated full-term pregnancies.

She laments on the lack of funding for this disease even though it is the most common genetic disorder for babies. She is disappointed with the type of care that sickle cell patients receive. They are often treated as drug seekers, and even Black doctors are reluctant to prescribe them the narcotics they may need due to concern about being over-prescribers of narcotics. She believes there needs to be a pipeline to encourage more doctors to pursue management of this disease.[15]

Dr. Megan Clowse is an Associate Professor of Medicine in the Division of Rheumatology and Immunology at Duke University School of Medicine and the founding director of the Duke Lupus Clinic.[16] She has published extensively on the impact of lupus on pregnant women. She has helped to establish a program to educate healthcare providers on lupus. Inspired by her dedication, I wanted to learn more. She graciously spoke with me, with only a few days' notice, even though we had never met.[17] Even before she went to medical school, Megan Clowse had an interest in the health of women and families. In her undergraduate years at Johns Hopkins University, as part of her senior thesis as a history of science major, she focused on the origins of the birth control pill and the relationship with the Planned Parenthood in Baltimore, where she worked. She then pursued a master's in public health with a focus on population and family health. During medical school, she realized that she was not interested in the field of obstetrics and gynecology and was fascinated by the field of rheumatology. She thought her service to women's health was largely behind her. Little did she know that it was just beginning.

She was in her first month of training as a rheumatology fellow, also at Johns Hopkins University, when she was called to consult on the labor floor. At first, she did not even know where it was located since she had never needed to go there before. The patient was a young Black woman at about 20 weeks of pregnancy, her third pregnancy. She had the rare complication of only having severe lupus flares during pregnancy, and it presented a treatment dilemma for her medical team. Working with the high-risk obstetricians, Dr. Clowse and her colleagues needed to decide on the best and safest drugs for their mutual patient. The patient was given two drugs that were not likely to have had any adverse effects on her developing baby. However, within two days her baby had died. Six months later, having never left the hospital, the patient also died. The impact on Dr. Clowse was significant. She wanted to learn more about her former patient's medical history and wanted to find a way to save other women like her. With access to the work of great researchers at her institution, she was able to gain an increased understanding of the problem, but she did not learn how to fix it. Her work was not over.

At the same time, she was undergoing a difficult journey in her personal life. She was facing difficulties getting pregnant. When she finally did get pregnant, she was forced to be on bedrest for four months. The personal and professional merged in a way she had not expected, and her commitment to the reproductive health of women and pregnancy care for women with rheumatologic conditions was strengthened. Thankfully, despite being born at 32 weeks, her daughter did well.

Dr. Clowse carried this passion to Duke University at a time when the only way to advance her work was to be an innovator, since few others recognized its value. A grant from the National Institutes of Health made her work and her research possible. During those years, her personal life collided with her professional life once again. She became pregnant with her second child and had an uncomplicated pregnancy. Her path again diverged from the routine when her son, after being delivered by a repeat cesarean section, did not breathe. A breathing tube was placed, and specialists were enlisted to determine the cause of his symptoms. The baby was diagnosed with a rare condition, and Dr. Clowse and her husband were told that the expected outcome was his death. They refused to accept that fate for their child. Research revealed that a small number of children survived. Nine and a half weeks later, their son was one of those. As suddenly as his condition appeared, it has resolved; and having recovered, he was sent home. Dr. Clowse and her husband were given the joy of raising their children, both of whom are now in their teenage years.

During those many bleak, uncertain days in the hospital, a pediatric colleague visited with Dr. Clowse and her husband daily. The colleague was showing compassionate support for his friends: his own wife who had been under the care of Dr. Clowse and was also a dear friend had successfully given birth to children despite a debilitating rheumatologic condition. About a year after Dr. Clowse's son was born, her colleague's wife had succumbed to her disease. Her parting words were shared in a letter read at her funeral. She wrote of the joy her children brought to her life, despite the pain of living with a debilitating illness. She wrote of her children making her life worth living. Her second passion was her work. She enjoyed her work and fundamentally believed one's work should have a positive impact on the world.

To Dr. Clowse, the message was loud and clear, even if she had any doubt prior to that time, she knew with absolute certainty that her life's mission was to help women with rheumatologic diseases have the children they desire, as safely as possible. She knew that their pregnancies would not always be perfect; she knew that the outcomes would not always be perfect, but neither were hers. Being imperfect does not mean being less valuable. Dr. Clowse works to counteract the medical biases against women with difficult rheumatologic conditions who choose to have children. She works to counteract the racism that Black women with these conditions continually face. She has come to believe that diseases of predominantly Black women are not sufficiently supported by research and investment, and, as such, it is the reason why the care in conditions such as lupus is so far behind. She recognizes that in many emergency rooms, lupus patients are mistreated and treated as drug-seeking patients, many living at the intersection of being Black and being women. These patients are not believed because they are one or the other, or both. When they become pregnant, the treatment gets even worse.

"So much of what is wrong is a social construct with racism being a huge part." Dr. Megan Clowse is a part of the solution.

Black pregnant women with conditions such as SCD and lupus magnify the health disparities for Black pregnant women in multiple ways. Lack of investment in the conditions lead the women to enter pregnancy not only ill informed, but with serious deficiencies in medical readiness. This underfunding further exacerbates the lack of expertise when caring for them during pregnancy. Expertise that is often tainted by biases, both explicit and implicit. Investments are not only needed to advance the knowledge of caring for these women, but to recruit and retain healthcare professionals, including those who not only provide hands-on patient care but devote their time to research to develop or advance therapeutics. Professionals who, like Dr. Francis-McBarnette from yesteryear or Dr. Bronté-Hall and Dr. Clowse from today, recognize that their role is more than just a job: it's personal.

I believe that Connie was treated with dignity in the days leading up to her death. I believe my colleague did everything she possibly could to save her. I don't know if her care was limited by the absence of state-of-the-art equipment or medication. When I think of Claudia, my thoughts diverge. I do think she may have had access to state-of-the-art equipment and medication but, by her own words, she was not treated with dignity and respect; and I will always wonder if the doctors did everything they could to save her.

CHAPTER 12

Mental Health Challenges— The Silent Pandemic

While I think I have an animated personality, I am usually pretty good at keeping my emotions in check in professional settings. Even if I am feeling particularly sad, angry, or upset, I have been able to maintain a pleasant face and upbeat demeanor for my patients and others. But I am not perfect. I remember noticing displays of emotions from surgeons, predominately White males, when I was in training. I don't remember tears or sadness, but anger; frustration, if the surgery was not going well or if the necessary equipment was not in the operating room. Often, the outbursts were met with a scurry of activity by the nurses and other operating-room staff to get the surgeon what he needed.

In residency, a more-senior resident was particularly hard on me. It was within my first two years, already difficult for many reasons, and I had expected her to be an ally, but she was not. One day, my emotions got the better of me. We were behind closed doors, and I expressed myself in anger. I don't recall anything I said, but I know I raised my voice.

Unfortunately, someone overheard. He was the Chief Resident of Pediatrics at the hospital I was rotating through. He was a White male from Germany. He offered immediate compassion. I had been rotating on his team for a few weeks. He said, "Monique, I know that is not you, what happened." I offered a few details that I felt comfortable sharing, and we moved on. He never brought it up again. He never treated me differently. I will never forget his compassion.

I rarely get angry in a professional setting. If I have, it has been either out of concern that my patient is not getting essential care that she needs or, even more rarely, if I have had to tolerate a certain behavior from a colleague and was not able to work through the issue. It is often compounded by other stressful professional circumstances. In the two other instances that I recall, I was never met with that level of compassion. I was reminded of my failures on one occasion months after I had apologized. That's part of what it is like to be a woman in America, particularly if you are a Black woman in the workplace, according to a *Harvard Business Review* article investigating the "Angry Black Woman" stereotype.[1] Emotions, such as anger, expressed by Black women are less often met as a reaction to an external circumstance, usually accorded to non-Black people or even Black men, but as a personal character flaw. The authors shared two studies which confirmed this finding. It is not that these expressions of anger are necessarily OK or appropriate; it's just that Black women are judged more harshly for expressions that are simply human.

Maybe at least partially due to this harsh judgment, many Black women in America have learned to silence their emotions and appear as the "Strong Black Women," which causes further negative impacts on their mental health.[2] However, judgment does not necessarily only come from outside the Black community. When I was growing up in Jamaica, I certainly didn't notice mental-health problems being given the same status as other health-related problems. If someone had a mental-health problem, it was discussed quietly, secretively. When I was told someone had a "nervous breakdown," I felt that a personal weakness was implied. I have never felt that implication with, for example, hypertension, diabetes, or cancer. Frankly, in many circles, this has been the same in the United States. I have only noticed changes recently, especially with the bravery of young Black female athletes such as Naomi Osaka and Simone Biles being open with their struggles.

What does that mean for Black women in the pregnant and post-partum period? A systematic review published in 2016 found that, in the majority of studies they reviewed, non-Hispanic Black women were more likely to have depression compared to non-Hispanic White women during pregnancy.[3] The prevalence of depression, which ranged from 10% to 30%, was determined by any of three factors, including being diagnosed by a physician, self-reported depressive symptoms, or determined to have depression by a depression-screening tool. Furthermore, the researchers found that for Black women there was a correlation between depression and a history of abuse, a higher number of children, lower self-esteem, and higher stress. Despite the evident need of Black women for mental health treatment, another study has shown that Black women are less likely to receive mental-health treatment than White women, even after accounting for multiple factors including age, education, marital status, income, employment, and health insurance.[4]

Earlier in my career, I don't recall diagnosing many pregnant women with depression or any other mental health disorder. The problem is there was not much in place for me to be able to make such a diagnosis. I would have had to rely on a patient telling me she had a problem while asking for help.

Apart from a psychiatry rotation in medical school, I recall little, if any, further training in mental health during my entire medical training. As I mentioned in chapter 7, in the context of discussing preeclampsia and other hypertensive disorders of pregnancy, when we, as physicians, are well trained to recognize a certain condition, then we can be better at diagnosing it in a timely manner and getting our patients treatment, the converse is also true. If we aren't as good at recognizing a condition, we won't be as good at diagnosing it. This might at least partly explain the findings of another research study, which found that White women were more likely to be diagnosed and given medical treatment for depression than non-White women, including non-Hispanic Black and Hispanic women.[5] Even then, the rates of depression, as determined by diagnosis codes, were only 5.7% for White women and 2.9% for non-White women (including both non-Hispanic Black and Hispanic women)—substantially lower than the rates suggested by other studies.

What does this all add up to? Even though Black women may be more likely to experience symptoms of depression and other mental health conditions, they may be less likely to admit it than White women because of fear of how their concerns might be met by their physicians or other healthcare providers, or fear of stigma within the Black community. On the other hand, obstetrics and gynecology clinicians who generally do not have a lot of training in mental health are less likely to recognize it unless their patients bring it up and due to the multiple issues of bias, I have discussed, are even less likely to recognize it in their Black pregnant and postpartum patients. Where does that leave us?

Shortly after I returned to the United States in 2014, I noticed a change in mental health screening for pregnancy and postpartum women. This change likely resulted from the recommendations of the US Preventive Services Task Force that adults, including pregnant and postpartum women, should be screened for depression, with specific recommendations of screening tools that could be used.[6] My patients were receiving mental-health surveys, and I learned to look out for the results and review them. My diagnosis role became much easier. There were specific survey scores that would prompt me to refer a patient to get more help. Once she completed the survey, which was usually self-administered, I knew the recommended first step.

Unfortunately, that did not solve the entire problem. In some settings, I lacked the appropriate mental-health professionals to refer my patients to. An analysis completed by the Kaiser Family Foundation (KFF) reported that only 28.1% of areas in the United States have their mental-healthcare professional needs met.[7] While the report considered only psychiatrists and not the other groups of professionals, lack of mental-health professionals is still a problem.[8] Even if a professional were available, would they even be compassionate to the needs of my Black patients? The available research suggests that at least some might not be. Implicit negative bias against Black people pervades mental-health treatment, just as it does other areas of health.[9]

Frankly, even if the healthcare professional is caring and compassionate and free of the negative biases, some Black patients may be reluctant to trust them due to past trauma or other stigma associated with mental health. Taneasha White delves into some of those multiple issues in her article "Racism in Mental Health Care: Where Are We Now?"[10] She describes examples of disparities in the mental healthcare of Black patients, such as an increased likelihood of being given antipsychotic medication, being hospitalized without their permission, or being placed in isolation.[11] White highlights how implicit bias invades the care and discussions about the impact of racism on mental health. She includes real-life examples of how Black women, and other women of color, have been negatively affected in their access to necessary treatment or when they advocate for others in addition to the challenges of facing stigma in the Black community.

It is essential that we continue to screen for mental-health issues in all our pregnant and postpartum patients. It is also essential that we ensure that our Black patients have better access to culturally competent Black or non-Black mental-healthcare professionals. Adequate coverage needs to be provided by Medicaid, which as I have mentioned serves 65% of Black mothers,[12] and, of course, by private insurance. It shouldn't be the case that Black pregnant or postpartum women cannot get access to effective mental-health treatment because their insurance does not cover it, and if they cannot afford to cover the gap, that their needs are left unmet. Black women suffering from mental-health issues also need to feel supported by their respective Black communities.

Anger may be just an emotion, but it could also be a symptom of depression. According to a study published in 2018, anger can be present with symptoms of depression after a woman has a baby.[13] Additionally, postpartum women who experienced anger were more susceptible to other mental-health issues, such as anxiety and depression. Furthermore, mothers who had depression during pregnancy were more likely to report anger and hostility than women who only had depression after their babies were born. When mothers "had higher levels of depression and anger,"[14] their depression lasted longer.

The authors further commented that feeling powerless contributed to anger associated with postpartum depression. Feeling powerless and angry was associated with "economic hardship, relationship conflict and feeling trapped in current circumstances,"[15] conditions which I am certain, many Black women in America face.

While the available research does not suggest that Black women are more likely to have anger as a symptom of depression, or other mental-health condition in pregnancy and postpartum, the sad reality, based on my experience and those of many Black women, is that if they do have anger as a symptom, they may not be met with the compassionate care they need. All this does is make a bad problem worse.

I hope that in whatever capacity you work, or even in your private life, if you encounter a Black woman who exhibits anger, you display compassion, you give her the benefit of the doubt, like my chief resident did so many years ago. This can potentially begin to help her heal. If it is a larger mental-health problem, she may even feel safe enough to ask for help. I believe that this act of kindness and compassion will live on for many, as it has for me.

CHAPTER 13

Covid-19 and the Effect on Black Pregnant Women

Early in the Covid-19 pandemic, an ABC News contributor, Dr. Ayodola Adigun, reached out to me for my views on how the pandemic might affect Black pregnant women. Ever cautious with my words, I said: "it is perhaps not unreasonable to consider African American pregnant women at higher risk until proven otherwise."[1]

My cautiousness is based on the need to deliver accurate information, to the best of my ability, privately and publicly. Some of the CDC's missteps may have been based on similar values: trying to give accurate information at a time when too little was known about the virus to be completely accurate, and thereby either delaying sharing useful information or sharing guidelines that were not always practical to follow. While I did not have the public responsibility of the CDC, as an individual, I had to deal with an added layer. I knew that, as a Black physician, every word I uttered or shared publicly would be held to more intense scrutiny than statements by my White colleagues. Inadvertent mistakes might be pointed out in a "polite" email.

The truth is, I was much more certain than my words suggested. All my prior research and knowledge had informed me that Black pregnant women would be at a higher risk. Although race data is still inadequate, update after update has confirmed that Black and Hispanic pregnant women are more likely to develop serious complications and die due to Covid-19.[2] In the state of Mississippi, between March 1, 2020, and October 6, 2021, fifteen women died with a Covid-19 infection during pregnancy.[3] Nine, or 60%, of the women were Black. In the data, it is estimated that 43% of births are to Black women, but the racial makeup of the 1,637 infected pregnant women was not documented. It is interesting, however, that in most of the months of the documented deaths, the infection rate for White people was almost twice that for Black people, suggesting that this disparity is worse than what is suggested by the birth rate for Black women. The overall available data does not necessarily suggest that Black pregnant women are at a higher risk of contracting the disease.[4] However, in some states, they might be. A study out of Michigan found that Black pregnant women were twice as likely as White pregnant women to get infected with Covid-19.[5] Based on other information, which I described chapter 3 regarding the disproportionate number of Black women in low-income service jobs, it is plausible that this increased risk could be due to occupational exposures. Another study based on the same Michigan population also collaborated prior findings from a larger study that Covid-19 infection is associated with an increased risk of preeclampsia,[6] a condition which, as I have discussed in chapter 7, is already more prevalent among Black women. Furthermore, if the Black pregnant patients with Covid-19 developed preeclampsia, they were almost twice as likely as women of other races to deliver preterm, further adding to the burden they already had to bear.

Fortunately, unlike early in the pandemic, we now have vaccinations and treatments. But will they save Black pregnant women? We must do more than hope.

First, I want to discuss what else we have learned about the risks of the virus and the benefits of vaccinations for pregnant women: thankfully quite a lot. I have to thank the Journalist's Resource put out by Harvard Kennedy School for packaging this information very neatly.[7]

An analysis of more than 1.2 million deliveries that took place between March 2020 and September 2021 found that, overall, Covid-19 infection almost doubled the risk of a woman having a stillbirth, with the Delta variant being a strong contributor to that increased risk.[8] The likelihood of a stillbirth occurring was higher if the Covid-19 infections led to certain complications associated with severe disease, but it was also higher if the Covid-19–infected pregnant woman had chronic hypertension or a multiple gestation pregnancy.

What can put pregnant women at risk for severe illness?, you might ask. Fortunately, we have information on that as well. There are quite a few factors, including being twenty-five or older; having chronic lung disease (such as asthma), obesity, chronic hypertension, and diabetes; and working in places where it is difficult or impossible to be more than six feet away from someone who is sick. The severity of a woman's illness has correlated with the number of these preexisting medical conditions she faced: the more health conditions she had, the sicker she was likely to get.

As for the risk and benefits of vaccination specifically to pregnant women, the CDC and ACOG continue to accumulate data. The bottom line is that the vaccine protects pregnant women from more severe disease without increasing the risk of pregnancy-related complications beyond the usual rates. Complications which were specifically mentioned included gestational diabetes, hypertensive disorders of pregnancy, newborn (neonatal) death, preterm birth, and babies not growing at a normal rate in the uterus (intrauterine growth restriction, IUGR).[9]

Furthermore, studies have shown that protective antibodies are passed to the baby through the placenta and breastmilk (for lactating mothers);[10] and at least one study has shown that babies of mothers who were vaccinated during pregnancy were less likely to be hospitalized with Covid-19 infection during their first six months of life than babies of unvaccinated mothers.[11]

Despite the accumulative evidence of benefits with low risks, vaccination rates in pregnant women, and in particular Black pregnant women, remain low. A CDC report published in June 2021 examined the vaccine uptake among pregnant women in eight healthcare organizations for the period from December 14, 2020, to May 8, 2021. Only 16.3% of women had received one or more doses, but Black women were the least likely to have received at least one dose, with a rate of 6% compared to 19.7% for White women and 11.9% for Hispanic women.[12]

Part of the reason for the initially low vaccine uptake among pregnant women likely falls on the long-held, established practices in vaccine development, where pregnant women are deliberately excluded to avoid the potential liability risk if the vaccine conferred harm to the developing baby. The lack of information and uncertainty of risks have left pregnant women frightened and confused, even as prominent bodies, such as the Society for Maternal Fetal Medicine and ACOG, were quick to support the vaccination of pregnant women.[13] Early ambivalent statements from the World Health Organization (WHO) likely did little to combat the fears of pregnant women.[14]

While the most recent CDC data on the vaccination rates among pregnant women show improvement, the rates still lag behind the general population, and Black women remain even further behind. In the estimate reported on January 8, 2022, based on data from the Vaccine Safety Datalink, of all the women who were pregnant anytime from December 20, 2020, to January 20, 2022, and received at least one dose of Covid-19 vaccine, the rate was 43.2% for White women and 26.2% for Black women, including those who received the vaccine either prior to or during pregnancy, or both.[15]

I remember that, early in my counseling, I focused on explaining to pregnant women the potential life-saving benefits of the vaccine. Frankly, that was all we had. While we knew that there was no evidence of the vaccine being harmful to the developing fetus, supported by animal data, in the absence of trials in pregnant women, we could say little more.

The real problem with that line of counseling it is not what vaccine-hesitant pregnant women are interested in hearing.

A recently published review by a group of researchers based in Australia sought to answer that specific question: What factors were involved in the decision-making in vaccine-hesitant parents?[16] Three main themes arose. The first was vaccine safety: parents were concerned about bad reactions to the vaccine and the risk of long-term side-effects to them or their children.

The second major category was healthcare professionals: the information that healthcare providers shared with their patients highly influenced their decisions to accept vaccines; however, if healthcare professionals failed to provide the information to patients, or if patients felt their concerns were dismissed or needs ignored, then the opposite would occur.

Linked to this category was the important element of trust: if patients did not trust the healthcare professional—for example, as a result of, or exacerbated by, feelings that the healthcare professional dismissed their concerns or that the healthcare professionals were influenced by vaccine manufactures—then they would not want to accept vaccination.

The third category was alternative influences: if patients do not trust their healthcare professionals, then other sources of information become more important. This could include influences from family and friends or religious beliefs. However, a major factor was information people obtained from social media. It is well known that many conspiracy theories related to the vaccine were advanced on social media, and this has had a detrimental effect on vaccine uptake.

Another study published earlier in the pandemic shed some more light on factors which could affect women's willingness to take vaccines. This study specifically looked at pregnant women's willingness to take the flu or pertussis vaccine.[17] The likelihood of getting vaccinated was 10 to 12 times higher for women who had recommendations from their healthcare professionals; but if women believed the vaccine could cause them harm, they were five times less likely to be vaccinated. If pregnant women had more "general information" about the flu vaccines, or if they "knew there was a national vaccination policy in place," they were more likely to be vaccinated.[18] On the other hand, if pregnant women thought that the vaccine was unsafe in pregnancy or could cause birth defects or a miscarriage, they were less likely to accept the specific type of vaccine. If they believed the flu vaccine could provide benefits to them or their baby, or if they had a general sense of it being beneficial, they were more likely to be vaccinated.

But what do we know specifically about African Americans and other Black people in America as far as motivations about vaccine? First, let me state the obvious, which, unfortunately, sometimes is not all that obvious: Black people in America are not all the same. Differences are related to age, country of origin, socioeconomic status, the part of the country they live in, etc. So, clearly, any research to understand the vaccine uptake among Black people in America would be limited; however, I think there are some helpful findings.

One study examined the uptake of the flu vaccine in African American communities.[19] It specifically looked at vaccine behavior in the five year period prior to when the survey was administered in 2015. Vaccine knowledge which was correlated with increased age, income, and education was positively associated with the likelihood of getting a vaccine. Among the groups of African Americans, those who were never vaccinated (in that five year period) had lower trust levels, related to the Tuskegee Syphilis Experiment; those who were vaccinated against the flu once or twice within the past five years had the lowest income and had the greatest reported frequency and impact of discrimination. The lowest-income African Americans were also more likely to report using natural remedies rather than the flu vaccine.

What about Black pregnant women specifically? What factors affect their willingness to accept vaccines? Another study published recently examined the differences in attitudes of women of different racial groups toward being vaccinated in pregnancy.[20] It surveyed almost 2,000 women who were receiving their prenatal care from twenty-three practices in Georgia and Colorado from June 2017 until July 2018. The study evaluated the likelihood of White, Black, and Hispanic women to receive the tetanus, diphtheria and pertussis (TDAP) and flu vaccines, which are both routinely recommended in pregnancy. Black women were the least likely to intend to be vaccinated and more likely to be unsure about their vaccine intentions. They were less confident about the safety of the vaccine, less confident about the efficacy, and less likely to perceive the risk of vaccine-preventable diseases. Furthermore, they were less likely to report pro-vaccine social norms, perceive having enough vaccine knowledge to make a decision about infant vaccine choices, and trust vaccine information from healthcare providers and public health authorities.

I believe all this information not only gives us insight into why many Black pregnant women may be reluctant to get the Covid-19 vaccine, but also strategies to improve. I also think it shows that as much as people within and across racial and ethnic categories are different, frankly, what people need to convince them to take a vaccine is very similar: sound knowledge about vaccine risks and benefits and vaccine safety from a trustworthy source that respects their individual autonomy and decision-making skills.

Black pregnant women being less likely to be vaccinated is not a new problem, but in reading the research I really have to question how often, particularly low-income Black pregnant patients are being educated about vaccines when they are in the room with their health-care professional. Given the widespread presence of implicit bias in the community, I really wonder how many are given the time needed to discuss the risks and benefits of the vaccine in a non-judgmental and non-condescending manner. However, we would have to assume that healthcare professionals do know the risk and benefits of the Covid-19 vaccine, and frankly that is a big assumption.

A busy clinician seldom has time to keep up with the latest information on their own, so if this education is not incorporated into their workday or is not required learning, I can say with a great deal of certainty that many are less likely to know the information in depth.

If clinicians do not know detailed information or are not prepared to answer questions, it is less likely that they will be able to convince someone who is undecided.

The other matter is that patient visits are notoriously short. It may be enough time if patients have limited questions, and the pregnancy is low risk but of course that is not always the case and less so for many Black women.

Then, of course, there is the trust issue. Trust is built over time with mutual respect. If Black patients are allowed, as much as possible, to see their clinician of choice and that continuity is facilitated throughout the pregnancy, I am confident it will improve the trust and strengthen the uptake of recommendations by healthcare professionals, including vaccination. Healthcare institutions need to nurture the development of more clinicians of choice. As I have repeatedly mentioned throughout this book, the workforce needs to be better trained to address the needs of their Black patients in an empathetic, non-judgmental manner. Those who excel in patient care, as determined by patient perception and outcome, should be rewarded both financially and with increased flexibility of time. In multiple settings, I've seen just the opposite: their patient load is increased, and that leads to increased burnout, which in turn diminishes not only the quality of care but also the compassionate manner in which the healthcare professionals are able to deliver it.

Covid-19 is just another lens on the disparities Black pregnant women face. In the system as it exists today this was inevitable. Similarly, the vaccination rate among Black pregnant women is a disproportionate problem because, collectively, healthcare and we as healthcare professionals have not provided the knowledge or care that Black women deserve and consequently have failed to earn their trust. Nevertheless, all the solutions are in our hands—we just need to implement them.

CHAPTER 14

The Route of Delivery

I remember it like it was yesterday, even though it was 2008. Our first son Zane was born just over a month before the United States of America elected its first Black president. The labor pains started as mild cramps about five o'clock in the afternoon. My years of training helped me to quickly recognize it for what it was. By 8 p.m., three hours later, the contractions got progressively more frequent and stronger. Some relatives came to visit us at our family home in Florida. *Dancing with the Stars* was on television, and my parents were in the living room entertaining. I wanted to be polite and went in and out of my room. I didn't want to advertise the fact that I thought I was in labor, but I needed peace and quiet, so I contacted my doctor and I asked my husband to take me to the hospital. My doctor—one of my colleagues from my first job out of my obstetrics-and-gynecology residency—was a close and trusted friend.

My contractions were about five minutes apart, and every bump on the short fifteen-minute ride to the hospital was especially painful. I remember thinking how I had blithely given out instructions to my patients, maybe hundreds of times before, to come to the hospital when their contractions were five minutes apart, with a complete lack of awareness of how painful that ride must have been.

When I was settled in the triage room, the nurse checked me. I was 6 centimeters; an expecting mother generally starts to push when her cervix is dilated to 10 centimeters. I felt proud that I had gotten to 6 centimeters (the active phase of labor per ACOG criteria[1]), without the assistance of any pain relievers. My colleague arrived shortly after.

He checked me, but it was not good news. He determined that I needed a cesarean section. My cervix was swollen, and the tip of my baby's head already had detectable signs that it might have been a struggle to get through, something called caput. It is the swelling of the baby's scalp, more often associated with long labors.[2] I was deeply disappointed, but I trusted him and readily agreed.

My anesthesia was administered by a certified registered nurse anesthetist, someone whom I also knew and trusted, but another problem occurred. Despite signs to suggest my spinal anesthesia was appropriately given, I felt pain. Surely this cannot be normal. My patients rarely reported such pain to me when I had performed the procedure so many times before. My doctor listened and I was given additional anesthesia. It was yet another personal reminder of the importance of listening to my patients when they tell me that they are in pain.

I went to sleep and missed the entirety of my first birth experience. I will never have the memory of my son's first moments of life. Those moments are gone forever. Another lesson for me, and reason to assist and encourage patients to avoid general anesthesia (being put to sleep) whenever possible; but sometimes, as in my case, there is no choice.

Fortunately, my husband was allowed to remain in the room. He was able to film our son's first moments of life and capture the moment when our son was brought to me (a moment that I would never have any recollection of). Three hours later, at about 3 a.m., I saw my son for the first time. The nurse brought him to the room and told me he was hungry. Thankfully, the circumstances of the surgery did not compromise my ability to successfully breastfeed my first-born, another priority for me. Neither did it compromise my ability to bond with my first born. This is not true for every woman. One of my high school classmates shared that she believes her cesarean delivery thwarted her ability to bond with her child in the earliest days, a painful memory that has stayed with her.

Later that day, my doctor—my colleague and friend—came to check on me. Immediately sensing my disappointment with my route of delivery, he explained it in detail. Intellectually, I knew he was right. But I also knew that the possibility of me ever having a vaginal delivery had all but disappeared. I was already of advanced maternal age (age thirty-five or older in the obstetric world), and despite the absence of other

risk factors, it was a time when few (including myself) felt comfortable allowing a vaginal birth after cesarean section (VBAC) trial in a
community hospital.

My mother delivered all three of her children by cesarean section as
well. In her case, her first cesarean followed several hours of pushing to
attempt a vaginal delivery. My colleague had essentially saved me from
that ordeal; the pointed swollen head and puffy eyes of my newborn
were a testament to the likely outcome, hours of pushing and still
ending up with a cesarean section.

The ability to perform a cesarean section can be life-saving for both
mother and baby, but like almost any good thing, it can be misused or
abused. Not all of us, as obstetricians, are equally conscientious in its
use, equally skilled in its application, or equally knowledgeable in its
indication. It appears on all three parameters, Black women in America
are more likely to get the short end of the stick.

Black women have more cesarean deliveries than any of the racial
groups identified, with a rate of 35.9% compared to 30.7% for White
women, based on 2018 to 2020 averages;[3] and while this includes repeat
cesarean sections, other data looks no better. Black women in America
who are having their very first baby at full term, with the baby in
the correct position for vaginal birth, (head down, or cephalic), and
carrying only one baby, are more likely to have a cesarean section than
White women. In 2020, the rate was 30.6%, compared to 24.9% for
White women,[4] a trend that continues to worsen instead of improve.

Yet the current trends for cesarean section rates for Black women
seem to defy the original intentions of this surgery since neither mother
nor baby appear to be better protected by the practice.[5] Even a scheduled repeat cesarean section has more risk than if a woman is able to
successfully have a vaginal birth after a cesarean (VBAC).[6] Just ask
Charles Johnson who, after his wife Kira died following a scheduled
C-section, has become a tireless advocate to improve maternal care.

I mentioned Kira Johnson's death in the introduction to this book
and in chapter 4. What I did not mention is Charles Johnson's testimony.[7] He describes the hours of watching his wife's health deteri-
orate. He describes the multiple times he begged the medical staff
for help. He describes being told by the staff that his wife was "not
a priority." He describes the moments before his wife's return to the

operating room where she shared with him that she was scared. He explains how he worked, "doing everything in his power" to remain calm and keep his wife reassured. He recalls the doctor telling him, just before the surgery, that he would get to see Kira in fifteen minutes, but he never did see his wife, his best friend, the love of his life alive, ever again.[8] Charles Johnson is so confident that his wife died because she was a Black woman, that racial discrimination led to her death, that he filed a civil-rights lawsuit against Cedars-Sinai, the hospital where his wife had her baby and then died.[9]

The cesarean section rates aren't equal for every hospital in a particular state or between states. In fact, as I mentioned in chapter 4, studies show that in hospitals where Black women deliver, both Black and White women have a higher risk of birthing complications.[10] The quality of the hospital did not appear to be an issue for Kira Johnson who delivered in a nationally ranked hospital.

Being Black is one of the largest risk factors, leading to pregnancy complications that necessitate a cesarean section. These complications can be deadly, and the numbers are getting worse; but why? In 1996, the total cesarean section rate for Black women was 22%, which was only slightly higher than the rate for White women at 21%.[11] The maternal mortality rate in the United States was reported to be 7 to 8 per 100,000 live births for White and 18–22 for Black women.[12] By comparison, the rate for White women in 2020 was 19.1 deaths per 100,000 live births, versus 55.3 deaths per 100,000 live births for non-Hispanic Black women.[13] So the question is why is the rate of a procedure fundamentally designed to protect women and/or their babies increasing without making birthing safer for any woman in America and even worse for Black women?

While I have discussed other potential and proven causes for the negative trends in the Black maternal health throughout this book, I want to emphasize the relationship between the cesarean section rate and Black maternal morbidity and mortality more specifically.

To explain the overall change in use of cesarean sections, a little history may help. In 1996, I was in my second year of obstetrics and gynecology residency at Georgetown University Medical Center. My residency program director, Dr. Anthony Scialli, was a strong advocate for vaginal deliveries whenever possible, including allowing women the opportunity to have a vaginal delivery after a cesarean delivery—a position I quickly adopted, given my professional admiration for my teacher. Cesarean section rates in the United States were 21%,[14] impressively low compared to today's rates. I left residency in 1999, committed and passionate about ensuring that, if it is safely possible, women would have a vaginal delivery. However, the late 1990s, early 2000s in many ways marked the beginning of the end of one of the pro-vaginal delivery movements in the US obstetric world. In 1993, a paper published in the *American Journal of Obstetrics and Gynecology* discussed the rates of uterine rupture when a woman attempted a vaginal delivery after a cesarean section.[15] Among its key findings was something I incorporated in my counseling of women with a prior C-section who were attempting a vaginal birth. If more than 18 minutes pass between a prolonged drop in the baby's heartrate (as seen on the monitoring during labor) and delivery of the baby, the risks to the baby are significant.

In 1999 and 2001, the distinguished *New England Journal of Medicine* published two additional papers that further questioned the practice of allowing women to attempt vaginal births after cesarean sections. The first suggested that women should not be "mandated" to have a trial of labor after a cesarean section and that in certain settings a trial might be inappropriate.[16] The second discussed the rates of the uterus rupturing after a previous cesarean section and the additional risk posed by certain medications that were being used to help those women to go into labor.[17] In reviewing these three publications, it appeared that the push for vaginal delivery after a cesarean section was causing unnecessary harm.

Then in 2003 the American College of Obstetrics and Gynecology published an article about patient choice and cesarean section,[18] which, from my perspective as a newly minted fellow of ACOG, took things a step further. I interpreted the article as suggesting that a woman had the right to choose her route of delivery, and it was unethical to force her to undergo a vaginal delivery rather than a C-section, even if this was her first birth. In the years that followed I saw a trend in the number of women exercising that right. However, I suspect that in making that choice many of them did not know the possible consequences.

I vividly remember a woman coming into my private practice in the early years, shortly after this last article was published. It was her first pregnancy, and she insisted that she wanted a cesarean delivery. Having come from a pro-vaginal delivery background, I counseled her perhaps a little too adamantly to attempt a vaginal delivery. She ultimately agreed. Fortunately, she had a great outcome and continued to appreciate her vaginal route of delivery years later.

To be clear, regardless of the route, having a baby is not risk-free, but the goal of any obstetrician should be to deliver in a manner that maximizes the safety of both mother and child; and for the greater percentage of mothers that route is a vaginal delivery.

In 2015, the World Health Organization published a statement on the rates of cesarean section, where they specifically stated that above 10% there is no evidence that the mortality rates improve;[19] and while neither the WHO nor any other major organization agrees on what the "normal" rate is, many agree that the current rates are too high.

What are the risks associated with each of these routes of delivery for mother and child? In the short term, a C-section increases the mother's risk of multiple complications, including excessive bleeding at delivery, possibly requiring a hysterectomy, uterine rupture, wound complications, thrombotic events, and placental abnormalities, not to mention other complications of anesthesia and surgery. A C-section also poses risks to the baby, including increased risks of both short- and long-term respiratory problems, as well as a risk of the baby being cut inadvertently during the delivery.[20] Babies can also be at an increased risk of birth injury after a vaginal delivery, especially shoulder dystocia (a condition where the shoulders essentially get stuck after the delivery of the baby's head). Shoulder dystocia can lead to broken bones, temporary or permanent nerve damage; and the baby's oxygen supply could be severely compromised during the birth process. While the risk of this condition is low,[21] it certainly explains at least some of the reasons why cesarean sections are still needed. Cesarean sections may also reduce a woman's risk of urinary incontinence and pelvic organ prolapse.[22]

For Black women and their babies in America, it appears that all birth complications are magnified. One reason for this is that whenever Black women face complications, they are less likely to get the correct intervention in a timely manner. One would think that that would not apply to a superstar like Serena Williams; however, it did. Even when she had known risk factors for a complication that occurs more often after a cesarean section (the delivery route she underwent), she still had to be her strongest advocate.[23] Serena had a known history of blood clots and lived in fear of a recurrence. However, due to her surgery, she was off her daily medical preventative regime. When she felt short of breath, she made the immediate assumption that it was a pulmonary embolism (blood clots travel to the lungs, blocking the blood vessels and compromising vital blood flow). She walked out of her hospital room and informed the nurse that she needed a CAT scan and heparin (the diagnostic study and the medical treatment). The nurse initially dismissed her concerns, telling her that "all this medicine is making you talk crazy."[24] Serena did not give up, and her doctor was called and the necessary tests were ordered. She was able to get the life-saving medication and procedure she needed.

However, increased complication rates do not explain why Black women have the surgery so much more often now than in 1996. While there may not be an exact answer, there are certainly clues.

A few years ago, experts at Yale decided to look at the dramatic rise in C-sections rates that they noticed between 1996 and 2007, specifically because Connecticut, where the institution is based, had a greater than 70% increase in the rates.[25] While some of the increase was explained by women who had a C-section before and were getting another one, half of the large increase in rates was due to women having C-sections for the first time. Interestingly, some of the key reasons for the increase were conditions which sometimes, yet not always, necessitate cesareans, thus leaving room for interpretation and differences between physicians. For example, the leading reason for these procedures was something called "non-reassuring fetal status." Simply put, it is when the doctor thinks that the baby might be in trouble based on the monitoring of the baby on the fetal heart-tracing during labor. While it is often clear to most obstetricians when the monitoring looks very good or very bad, there is also a gray zone. While, as obstetricians, we might ultimately need to intervene and perform a cesarean section, the intervention is not required immediately, which could allow time for the baby to deliver vaginally. The Society of Maternal Fetal Medicine and various entities have put in a lot of work to help physicians improve their methods of interpreting fetal monitoring. Another big reason is something called "arrest of labor disorder." During arrest, a woman's labor seemingly stops. Research has come out to suggest that sometimes doctors decide to throw in the towel and do a C-section too quickly, while waiting a little longer might have allowed a vaginal delivery.[26] Another of the top five reasons for cesareans is preeclampsia; but preeclampsia is not in itself a reason for a C-section, and for reasons already discussed, it is more prevalent in Black women in America. I think that it is also worth mentioning that an 8% increase in C-sections was listed as being due to maternal request (simply put, women wanted to deliver via that route). While the races of women were identified in this study, race was not specifically discussed in relationship to the outcomes, so in my opinion this study provides only one piece of the puzzle.[27]

Researchers in California decided to look at the reasons why African American women were having more cesarean sections. They chose the year 2010 and looked at 255 California hospitals. They noticed that African American women were significantly more likely than the other races of women in the study to have C-sections, although they were no more likely than the other women to have a repeat cesarean section and at the time they were only slightly more likely to have had a previous C-section.[28]

African American women were more likely to have an elective cesarean section (by choice) and an emergency cesarean section. The researchers found that the risk factors that African American women had were not different when compared to those of other women, except that African American women were more likely to have a diagnosis associated with high blood pressure or preterm pregnancy and less likely to have a malpresentation (when a baby is not in the right position for a vaginal delivery).[29]

And yet, even though the likelihood of having a malpresentation (a less disputed indication for cesarean section) was lower for Black women, which could potentially have reduced the frequency of the surgery, Black women still had more C-sections. Notably, a fetal heart-rate abnormality was more likely to be diagnosed among African American women. Even African American women with no identifiable risk factors were still more likely to have had a primary C-section, elective C-section, or emergency C-section.

Having been an obstetrician for more than twenty-two years and recognizing the factors that go into a vaginal delivery, a few possible albeit somewhat controversial theories for the discrepancy come to my mind.

Waiting for a laboring woman to have a baby can take a great deal of time and patience. Since obstetricians likely have the same level of implicit bias as other health professionals (which is the same as everybody else),[30] it may be that those biases interfere with the desire to give their African American, or other Black, patients that time and patience, hence encouraging them maybe a little too soon to have the surgery. Or perhaps a lack of connection with the patient or concern that the patient does not trust them enough to be patient for a vaginal route leads them to jump to a C-section faster in order to ensure that the baby is delivered safe and sound. Similarly, Black women at the time of the study, up to 2010,[31] may have been more likely to believe that the best route of delivery for them was a C-section (possibly in a desire to keep their babies safe), especially since their babies are at least twice as likely to die than White babies. Their doctors may not have fully informed them of the risks of a cesarean section, again, because of that lack of connection.

The authors of the study suggest that "some women might have a cesarean recommended on the basis of their physician's misunderstanding their patient's pain threshold, articulated preferences, etc."[32]

In my career, I have had patients beg for cesarean sections due to the pain of labor. My solution is usually to improve their pain management and explain at length that pain is not a reason for the surgery. When that same demand is made to many doctors, are some less likely to give that lengthy explanation to Black women?

Apart from the factors above, it appears that there are specific factors in the birthing experience that may literally make healthy Black pregnant women sick, to the point of affecting their fetal tracing, and ultimately affecting their delivery outcome, leading to even more C-sections. As I discussed in the introduction, it has now been shown conclusively that the chronic effects of racism are negatively affecting the health of Black women and causing their biological age to exceed their chronological age. Could it be that racism in labor is causing short-term stress reactions that lead to an increase in fetal tracing abnormalities?

Actress Tatyana Ali might say yes. She candidly described her first birthing experience in an article for *Essence*, an experience which left her "traumatized."[33] She wrote that despite multiple people being in her delivery room, she felt that no one was there to really help her. Unfortunately, she felt that the lack of support included her doula who, she believes, had conflicting personal motives.

A recent study authored by Debbnick et al. and published in 2022 appears to further strengthen at least some aspects of my hypothesis.[34] As suggested by the previous study, Debbnick et al. showed that low risk non-Hispanic Black women who had never given birth were again more likely to undergo a C-section than similar non-Hispanic White women with the rate being 22.8% compared to less than 18%. It probably isn't a surprise that the only indication for the surgery that occurred more often for Black women was, you guessed it, non-reassuring fetal status. But, as a physician and someone acquainted with multiple physicians who are dedicated to giving each and every patient optimal care, I know there is more to the story.

An argument is made to increase midwifery care in hospitals. Research has shown that low-risk patients under the care of midwives had approximately 30% lower risk of having a cesarean section if this was their first delivery, and 40% lower if they had delivered prior to that time.[35] They were also less likely to have an operative delivery (i.e., when a device such as a vacuum or forceps are used to help the baby deliver). On the negative side, patients who had prior deliveries were more likely to have shoulder dystocia when cared for by midwives.

However, the percentage of African American women who participated in the study was less that 5%, and the study therefore did not specifically examine the impact of midwifery care on the C-sections rates for Black women. Furthermore, some studies do not corroborate that midwifery care lead to lower C-section rates.[36] While more midwifery care could still be beneficial in the United States, just as in the case of physician care, if the midwife is non-Black and/or not culturally sensitive, this intervention may do little to lessen the disparities for Black women.

A hospital birthing experience is not only dependent on the doctors or midwives but in many ways more highly dependent on the bedside nurse. The nurse is usually with the mother for 8 to 12 hours of labor, depending on the nursing shift and the length of a mother's labor. The cultural sensitivity and the case load of that nurse can have a significant positive or negative impact on that outcome. If a nurse is culturally sensitive, well trained, and is not expected to manage an excessive number of laboring patients, she can provide the support the patient needs to optimize the outcome.

Over my career spanning almost twenty-five years post training, I have worked with many nurses. After a relatively brief interaction I can often make a reasonable assumption on the dedication and experience of the nurse, and I have seen my assumptions play out in the course of a patient's labor and delivery process.

The nurses who stand out for me are key supporters of the patient by not only ensuring that the patient's physical needs are met, including food, drink, pain management, and even a shower, but also that the labor is progressing normally and that appropriate intervention when needed is delivered in a timely manner. I believe that some of those outstanding nurses were integral to assisting some of my patients in having successful vaginal deliveries. Because physicians may not always be in the hospital, and when we are, we may have other duties, nurses keep us informed of the progress of the patients and can nudge us to initiate simple interventions that can enhance a patient's chance of success. With nursing shortages, frequent staff changes at hospitals, increasing use of travelers who, despite their qualifications, may not be as familiar with the culture of the hospital, quality nursing support appears to be happening less often even for White patients; and for Black patients, negative biases are added into the mix.

The bottom line is that the clinicians who deliver the babies are not the only people we have to be concerned about or who need "fixing." Beyond the delivering clinicians and nurses, the aesthetics of the delivery room, any other support staff who come in, including residents and students, if applicable, all play a role in the experience. How cohesive is the team, and, most importantly, are we able to place our patients at the center of our decision-making regardless of their color or any other factors that might trigger our bias? The sad reality in America today is that the answer is negative for too many Black women.

I had the pleasure of delivering many babies during the first year of the pandemic. Serving a diverse practice, my patients were of multiple races and ethnicities, and while I always attempt to establish a bond with all my patients, I remember a particular Southeast Asian couple who stood out for two main reasons: the delivery went particularly smoothly, and the husband had a doula on the phone the entire time. But the benefits of doula support are not just anecdotal which I discussed at length in chapter 10. Frankly, for many Black mothers in America, doulas may be key to keeping the woman safe during the delivery process.

Since system change can take years, Black women do not have time to wait, given the dire situation that they are in regarding their maternal health. Each Black patient should be given (at a minimum) doula support when they are in labor, if they do not already have one during their pregnancy. Since the connection with, and motivations of, the doula matter, expecting parents should be allowed to interview and choose the doula they use and be provided with resources to facilitate their choice. Fortunately, resources are available through entities like the National Birth Equity Collaborative to help with the choice. If hospitals, clinics, and practices provide Black women with information about doula resources, and insurance companies, including Medicaid, finance doula services, the cost-saving potential could be significant. And we can do even more to improve outcomes and reduce C-section rates for Black women. On a system level, we need to ensure that culturally appropriate education about the pros and cons of the route of delivery is given to Black women and stop assuming that one size fits all in the education that's delivered. Black women with high levels of education may be further harmed by assumptions that their health literacy is limited, and Black women with lower levels of education may also be harmed by attitudes that they will be unable to comprehend their options.

The health system needs to ensure that the skill of the clinician matches the labor needs of the patient, and knowing that Black patients are more at risk for cesarean sections, the adequacy of staffing for their labor management should be considered.

Telehealth capabilities could be used to support clinicians who work in underserved settings. Sometimes all they need is another physician (even remote) to review and discuss the interpretation of an ambiguous fetal-heart tracing. The wishes of Black patients, like those of all patients, should be respected throughout the course of their labor and delivery, and open communication should be maintained throughout the process.

Clinicians who are deemed to support culturally sensitive care should be rewarded in manners that have been shown to be effective, to not only enhance their likelihood of continuing to deliver such care but to encourage others. Of course, this should supplement rather than replace any initiatives that are already in place.

In 2014 the American College of Obstetrics and Gynecology published a document entitled the Safe Prevention of Primary Cesarean Delivery.[37] This document which was reaffirmed in 2019 reviewed the scope of the problem and included evidenced-based approaches to attempt to improve clinician decision-making when determining the need for a cesarean section. The California Maternal Quality Care Collaboration (CMQCC) put words into action and launched a "multi-faceted, multilevel initiative,"[38] which successfully reduced the rate of cesarean section of first-time low-risk birth mothers from 26% in 2014 to 22.8% in 2019 without any evidence of worsening outcomes for the babies. However, unfortunately, this study did not specifically look at variables affecting Black women, so clearly more work needs to be done.[39] The CMQCC has acknowledged its "past misalignment of strategies" and has expressed its commitment to birth equity.[40]

As an obstetrician, I am thankful that I have the option of offering women a safe C-section when needed. Many times, over the course of my career, I have had to perform one, sometimes within minutes, to save a baby's life. I remember many of these experiences vividly. I shudder to think of the consequences if this were not possible. I am grateful to have my two healthy children who were delivered by C-section. Initially, I was disappointed, since it was not my desired route of delivery, but the disappointment was short-lived because of my confidence in my doctor. I knew he made the very best decision for both me and my children. However, this potentially life-saving surgery needs to be used appropriately for all women, and Black women should not be excluded. Each and every Black woman who delivers in America, like any other woman, regardless of her race, religious beliefs, or ethnic background, should be given clear guidance about the recommended route of delivery so that together she and her clinician can make the very best choice.

CHAPTER 15

The Postpartum Experience—The Care That Ends Too Quickly

About twenty-four hours after delivering my son, I began shivering uncontrollably and felt intense pain. "What is happening to me?," I thought. Was it a fever? Did I have an infection? I alerted my husband, who remained at my bedside throughout my hospitalization. We decided to call the nurse. She came in and quickly reassured me that it was just the spinal anesthesia wearing off. I felt silly. I had already been an obstetrician for almost ten years at the time, but I didn't recall learning about this side-effect. It was another reminder of all those patient experiences that are not seen when I wear my physician hat. Otherwise, my hospital stay was relatively uneventful. In some ways, it was enjoyable: I had all my meals provided, and my obligations were limited to feeding myself and my baby. Additionally, I had key breastfeeding support from the lactation consultants. However, I did have a visit from a Special Supplemental Nutrition Program for Women, Infants, and Children (WIC) representative. WIC is a supplemental nutrition program for women, infants, and children offered to economically disadvantaged women. I am a big fan of WIC, as it is an excellent resource to help to provide healthy food to women and children who would have considerable difficulty affording it for themselves. Multiple studies have shown the benefits of WIC participation for maternal and child outcomes. The benefits include reductions in the number of low-birthweight and very-low-birthweight babies, reductions in preeclampsia, reductions in preterm birth and perinatal death.[1] In 2008, when my first child was born, to qualify for WIC, a household of four would have to have a combined income of less than $40,000 per year. At the time of the visit, the only thing I knew was that it was a benefit provided to economically disadvantaged mothers and children.

I found myself wondering: do all patients at this hospital—including doctors—get this visit (because that would seem like a waste of resources), or did I get this visit because I was Black? I never asked that question of the WIC representative, but it is far too easy to recall the negative emotions their visit elicited. Was it assumed that just because I was Black, I could not possibly be able to feed my child without additional financial support? I felt offended. As I ponder this experience, I realize that the same negative emotions that I felt being offered WIC could be true for my Black patients, regardless of their income level. The negative emotion could potentially lead some low-income Black patients to refuse much-needed help only to avoid being stereotyped. My experience could have been different: if the WIC representative had come into my room and said that it was standard hospital procedure that all women delivering babies are educated about WIC, I would have listened. I would have learned. I would have asked questions. I would have gained vital information to share with my patients. Instead, I remember the experience as an example (albeit minor) of the negative bias that African American women have to face throughout their entire lives—a bias that I was not only spared in the developmental years I spent growing up in Jamaica, but in much of my pregnancy which was also spent in Jamaica.

I also experienced really outstanding and positive postpartum care. One example was my interaction with a patient care assistant. She was a young Asian woman who was working in that capacity with hopes of pursuing further studies in healthcare. She carefully helped me to remove my dressing as painlessly as possible, because she knew it would hurt. Caring hospital staff matter, regardless of their position.

I am also grateful for the care I received during a rounding visit from a physician colleague. He was also one of my former partners from my first job. I was considering going home the evening of my second day after surgery. He encouraged me to remain another day: "Nothing good about going home at night." His words impacted my care delivery ever since, and I avoid as much as possible the practice of sending home new mothers in the evening, which unfortunately is sometimes required for mothers with limited medical coverage. The problem is that they may be sent home to an environment with a limited supply of food, limited social support, or to an environment where they may have to immediately assume childcare responsibilities for other children, regardless of the fact that they have barely begun healing from their delivery. I returned home the following day, instead.

I had plenty of support from my husband, my younger brother, and my parents. Nevertheless, it was overwhelming: the pain from my C-section, what appeared to be almost constant demands of breast-feeding, combined with concerns about whether my milk supply was sufficient, and a newborn that seemed to awaken constantly at night. When my husband had to return to Jamaica, leaving me to follow a few weeks later, things got even worse.

I shudder to think of the additional stress on women who have even less support and less knowledge of the post-delivery course.

Despite the loving support of her mother Wanda, Dr. Shalon Irving also felt overwhelmed after giving birth. But the stress of new mother-hood was compounded by serious health conditions including hypertension; a health condition that made her more likely to experience blood clots; a wound complication which involved multiple dressing changes; and multiple persistent and worrying symptoms, which made her know something was wrong.[2] Shalon and her mother did their best to seek care and to alert their healthcare providers. But the multiple visits and cries for help were not enough when it came to aiding yet another Black woman. They weren't enough even though this Black woman worked for the CDC, had two PhDs from a well-respected tertiary institution, had excellent health insurance, and likely received care from a reputable practice. It did not matter. Three weeks after having her baby, Shalon collapsed. Only a few hours before she collapsed, she had a clinician visit, a last desperate attempt to get the care she needed. She was prescribed blood pressure medication and was told to just give her symptoms "more time."[3] I am hard pressed to believe that she was given the comprehensive care she needed to ensure that she would have time to enjoy the life of her beautiful daughter, Soleil. Her autopsy showed that she died from complications of hypertension.

Fifty-two percent of maternal deaths occur in the postpartum period,[4] about 19% in the first six days after delivery, 21% between seven and forty-two days, and 12% from forty-three days to a year after birth. Overall, about 60% of these deaths are preventable. Among the leading causes of death in the first six days after delivery are hypertensive disorders, which I have discussed in chapter 7. Between forty-three days and one year (the late postpartum period), women are more likely to die from a condition called cardiomyopathy. Black women are more likely to die within the late postpartum period than White women, and cardiomyopathy is believed to be the most likely reason for this disparity.

Cardiomyopathy is basically a group of conditions where the heart muscles do not work well, and as a result they become less effective at pumping blood through the body.[5] Cardiomyopathy can lead to heart failure and death. Some of the symptoms are shortness of breath, fatigue, and swelling in the arms and legs. The interesting thing about these symptoms is that they are common symptoms of pregnancy. If a Black pregnant or postpartum patient sees her healthcare professional because her knowledge of her body and of herself tells her that her symptoms are not normal pregnancy symptoms, but she is ignored, disbelieved, or dismissed, she can die. Hypertension, especially if not properly treated, can lead to cardiomyopathy, heart failure, and death.

To be clear, even the best obstetricians and gynecologists may have a limited understanding of these conditions, but we must be the gatekeepers to ensure that we refer women with these conditions to get timely, appropriate care. We need a network of clinicians, including cardiologists, to refer patients to, and cardiologists need to ensure that our patients get all the care they need.

Based on the extensive report by Nina Martin in her brilliant *Propublica* series,[6] and hearing Dr. Wanda Irving so eloquently tell her daughter's story, I have some ideas about what may have led to Dr. Shalon Irving's death. Martin's report discussed occasions where Shalon's blood pressure was dangerously high—high enough to warrant immediate intervention. However, my sense is that while the home-visiting nurse who initially obtained those high blood pressure readings may have been concerned, she may not have had the knowledge to realize that Shalon likely needed to go for evaluation immediately. Similarly, when Shalon's blood pressure showed improvement in the doctor's office the next day, the clinician may have felt a false sense of security. This was possibly compounded by implicit bias—a phenomenon, which I have described multiple times throughout this book—whereby healthcare clinicians give Black patients substandard care due to subconscious ideas they are not aware of. The sad reality is that many are still not aware, or don't believe, that the care they are giving to Black patients is substandard.

In Shalon Irving's case, as I mentioned in my TEDx talk in 2018,[7] this combination of factors, insufficient knowledge and implicit bias, may have sabotaged her ability to receive the adequate medical support she needed and prevent her death, even though she had no socioeconomic factors that would have otherwise limited her access to resources or specialists.

As I have already outlined, Medicaid insures 65% of Black women and 40% of births overall.[8] So even if a Black patient does not have to endure implicit bias or overt racism, even if a Black woman's initial care provider recognizes that she needs to be referred to a specialist for further care, that access might be limited because many specialists are less likely to accept Medicaid, or have limited access for Medicaid patients, compared to private insurance.[9]

For most of my career, the standard care for postpartum women was a follow-up visit at 6 weeks. If they had a C-section a 2-week incision check was added. For women with high-risk conditions the care was more individualized, but specific standards to follow were less easy to identify or keep up-to-date with. In 2018, ACOG, recognizing the need to reduce maternal morbidity and mortality, acknowledged that more care was needed and expanded the recommendation to "contact ... within the first 3 weeks postpartum" and "ongoing care as needed, concluding with a comprehensive postpartum visit no later than 12 weeks after birth."[10]

Basically, it seemed that the standard follow-up was, and is, no longer adequately supporting women. It may never have adequately supported Black women who have always had disparities in their maternal health outcomes, but now the gap appears to be widening. Furthermore, the recommended number of visits is lower than that suggested by the World Health Organization (WHO), which recommends at least four health contacts during the first 6 weeks.[11]

Theoretically, those increased visits could be a step in the right direction toward improving the postpartum care for women, but accommodating those visits is easier said than done. Compared to other developed countries, the United States has an overall shortage of clinicians providing obstetric care, and that includes both obstetricians and midwives.[12] I have witnessed this shortage both from a leadership position and as a physician delivering patient care. While additional resources are often invested in getting women into care during their pregnancy, those resources are often lacking after they deliver their baby. It seems like that care is left to the village surrounding the woman; except that for many women, this village does not exist.

If a woman has no health risk factors, she may be able to make it without the extra support, but that does not mean she is doing well without it. Years ago, I remember a 2-week post–C-section clinical visit from a patient who was under my care. She had delivered her baby earlier than expected and only had the support of her husband; her family, who lived overseas, was not yet able to visit her. I found her overwhelmed, fatigued, and though technically she had a normal exam, she was not doing well. Fortunately, I was able to recommend strategies, such as sleeping when the baby is sleeping, which she successfully implemented, and she was doing much better at her follow-up visit. But suppose she was someone who had a vaginal delivery and an unrecognized risk of postpartum depression? Having only one post-delivery visit at six weeks was standard of care at the time. What else could have happened in those 6 weeks?

Even if visits are available, some Black mothers may not be able to get to the clinic because of transportation difficulties or childcare responsibilities. The advice, "sleep when the baby is sleeping," may be just a fantasy if there are other young children to care for in the home.

Certain initiatives could help, and thankfully some have been implemented. The expansion of Medicaid benefits from the current sixty days up to twelve months postpartum through the American Rescue Plan, which was signed into law March 11, 2021, and came into effect April 1, 2022, could help.[13] Studies have already shown that expansion of those benefits can reduce maternal mortality when the effect was "concentrated among" Black mothers.[14] Nevertheless, states have to do their part for this to occur.

But how do we ensure that the well-trained clinicians are available for women to see? Entities that support Black women need resources to attract physician candidates to care for underserved women. While, to some degree, that already exists with loan repayment opportunities, too often talent is lost after the obligations are complete. From my personal observation, some of the reasons include less competitive salaries and excessive workloads. Patients seen in clinic settings often have multiple health risk factors, yet physician schedules are crammed with patients to ensure that the practice can maintain enough profitability even to keep its doors open. However, having insufficient time to care for high-acuity patients lends itself to overlooking or missing important health conditions or further compromising the patient–doctor interaction. A hurried and stressed physician is less sensitive to any patient's needs, and this problem is exacerbated by implicit bias. Many locations across the United States are being affected by the shortage of obstetricians, further limiting physician access for postpartum care.

Advanced practice practitioners (APPs) who have a more limited scope of practice are used to fill the gaps. Due to a lack of alternatives they may be compelled to see patients who are beyond the range of their clinical abilities, often with limited guidance. Additional efforts need to be focused on training APPs to have improved understanding and ability to handle the issues that postpartum women face with increased attention to problems faced by Black women who are most at risk. Additional support needs to be given to women who have high-risk conditions, and their care needs to be directed to clinicians with the appropriate training. Does the system ever get it right? Can Black women get the care they need in the postpartum period, care that sometimes means life or death?

Dr. Sally Ward* was a well-known physician in her community and throughout the hospital system. She was delighted when at thirty-two she became pregnant with her first child. She had strong family support and she was confident about being well cared for, even though she lived and worked in a predominantly White community, one of very few Black physicians. She began her care with a midwife, but after a 26-week scare with preterm contractions associated with large uterine fibroids, she transferred to an obstetrician who was comfortable with treating pregnant women with fibroids and delivering high-risk pregnancy care. Otherwise, her pregnancy was going well. She had normal blood pressures throughout; her diabetes screen was normal; she was normal weight at the start of pregnancy, and only gained the recommended amount during her pregnancy. She was induced two days before her due date, but after an eighteen-hour induction, her obstetrician determined that she needed a C-section as she failed to progress adequately in labor (meaning her cervix did not dilate sufficiently to allow a vaginal delivery). She described her surgical experience as "really good." Her very experienced doctor was assisted by another accomplished physician with almost forty years of experience. She went home three days after surgery with an uncomplicated hospital course. However, the day after discharge she noticed some changes. She wanted to take her baby for a walk, but she noticed her feet started to swell. She was surprised. She had worked in the hospital up until 39 weeks, constantly on her feet and her legs had never got swollen.

The next day, when she took her newborn to her family doctor, she commented on her swelling. He told her, "Calm down Sally, you're doing too much." She had a good relationship with her family doctor, and she knew he meant well. Later that night she mentioned to her husband that her feet started to tingle. He was also a physician and had a blood pressure machine available. He took her blood pressure and she saw immediate concern on his face. He insisted that they go to the hospital straight away. She knew the small-town emergency department had limited capabilities, but she did not want to journey an extra hour to her delivering hospital because she did not want to be so far from her newborn.

The emergency room was staffed by an APP who was the sole provider on duty that Saturday night. Her blood pressure was elevated there as well, and she was prescribed medications. She did not get a urine or blood test at that time, which are part of standard care when a recently postpartum woman comes in with new onset high blood pressure. Sally was sent home with an appointment to see her regular obstetrician three days later—the closest appointment that was available. She got home early Sunday morning and immediately started taking her medication. Monday evening, she developed a headache and started feeling fatigued. She asked her husband to recheck her blood pressure. From his grave reaction, she knew something was very wrong. He immediately took her back to the nearby hospital. It was again staffed by the APP she had seen two nights before. Her first blood pressure reading was 171/100; six minutes later it was 169/104. Sally's husband became exasperated: Why was she not being treated with antihypertensives? She tried to calm him by telling him she was OK. Only she was not. She was scared and sad. She was scared because she knew what the numbers could mean; scared that she might be another statistic. She knew the realities of maternal health outcomes for Black women in America. She was sad about leaving her baby, the new life who now mattered to her more than anything or anyone else.

The APP informed her husband that he was waiting to hear from the obstetrician. Her husband insisted: "You do not need to wait; her blood pressure needs to be treated." Per ACOG, acute onset systolic blood pressure over 160 in any pregnant or postpartum woman warrants expeditious treatment with antihypertensive medications. It took more than an hour for Sally to get all the treatment, which finally brought her blood pressure to a safer range. One hour and twenty-six minutes after she arrived it was 149/90. During that time, the obstetrician had been reached. The APP was instructed to immediately start magnesium sulfate, a medication used to prevent seizures, and to continue to ensure that the patient's blood pressure was treated. Sally was then transported by ambulance to her delivery hospital. It took three days for her blood pressure to be in a safe enough range that she could return home. Thankfully, she did return home, and both she and her baby continue to do well.

Dr. Sally Ward wonders if she should have been a better advocate for her own care the first time she went to the hospital, or whether her being a physician allowed things to be overlooked. Nevertheless, she knows that she is lucky. She wonders: what if her physician husband had not taken her blood pressure? What if he had not advocated for her treatment to be started? What if she did not have a nanny to leave her baby with? Would she had stayed at home despite her symptoms? What if it happened to someone who was not a physician, whose husband was not a physician? The problem is we know the answer.

Dr. Ward does not feel that her race had a negative impact on her care, but she is concerned about lack of knowledge. The APP was doing the best he could, but he did not have sufficient training to know how to care for her.

Postpartum is a difficult time at best, as mothers deal with the constant demands of their newborn, with sleep deprivation, emotional ups and downs, and pain from a delivery tear or a C-section. But it is so much worse if a mother has complications, so much worse if she has a chronic health condition that she has to continually treat. Healthcare professionals must be well trained to meet their needs not just in urban America but in rural America. Patient symptoms cannot be ignored or minimized, regardless of their race or social standing. America, we are failing our mothers in the postpartum period, but like almost every other time in their lives, we are failing our Black mothers even more.

CHAPTER 16

The Newborn Tax on Black Children

I love movies. Over the years I've watched all types. Well before I became an obstetrician, I remember actors (in the earlier years I only remember seeing males) announcing, "It's a girl" or "It's a boy" immediately after they delivered the babies. In all my years of practicing obstetrics, the baby's sex has never been the first thing I would notice. I look to see if the little body I'm holding is trying to move and I listen for that little body to cry. I almost hold my breath if neither occurs right away. Often, you have signs before the delivery that the baby might have some difficulty after being born. If it's a cesarean section or a preterm delivery, the pediatric team is almost always there. In both those cases, I hand the babies immediately to the team. They will make sure the baby is OK and allow the mother to see her baby as soon as possible. When it is a vaginal delivery, they are not always present. It's me and the nurse. We both have some basic training in newborn resuscitation. Some nurses have more experience and skill than others. I rely on those skills.

After I deliver a full-term baby vaginally, I usually place the healthy, moving, crying baby directly on its mother's abdomen, baby's skin against mother's skin. If the baby is not moving or crying, I look for the nurse or the pediatrician, or both, and hand the baby over to them. Everything must be OK. This mother's baby must be OK. But it is not always that way. Sometimes the baby needs help to breathe. Sometimes it takes only a few puffs of oxygen through a face mask. Sometimes a breathing tube needs to be placed. Meanwhile, I have to reassure the mother: "They are working on the baby; it will be OK." I don't dare to think that it won't be. But it's not always OK. Babies die. As obstetricians, we are more psychologically prepared if the newborn is very preterm, we know when the chances are low before delivery. If the baby is full-term, often we are not. We expect that the baby will be OK.

I don't believe that any mother can be fully psychologically prepared to see her baby die, whether her baby is born early or on time. Whether it's within hours after delivery or within months. Sometimes they die without warning. They die even when everyone thought they were fine.

Infant mortality is the death of a baby before his or her first birthday.[1] The rate is the number of infant deaths per 1,000 live births. In 2018, just under 6,000 Black babies were a part of the statistic.[2] To be clear, the tragedy of infant mortality does not have a color; the pain is no less real whether a mother is Black or White, whether she is Asian, Hispanic, or Indigenous American, or any other race or ethnicity. It's just that Black women suffer this tragedy more often than any other race of women in America. In 2018, that rate was 10.8, while the rate for non-Hispanic White women was 4.6.[3] The rates have gotten a bit better since I was shown the statistics in medical school, the awakening of my knowledge of the health disparities between Black and White Americans. In 1992, the rate was 6.9 for White babies and 16.8 for Black babies.[4] The rates have gotten better but the disparity, not so much. It was 2.43 then and in 2018 it was 2.35. America is generally getting better at taking care of their babies, especially those born prematurely but still not so much for Black babies.

In 2020, a somewhat disturbing study was published. The authors decided to examine whether or not the physician's being Black would affect the care of Black newborns. They examined 1.8 million hospital births in Florida between 1992 and 2015.[5] They discovered that when Black newborn babies were cared for by White physicians, they had 430 more deaths per 100,000 births than White newborn babies. However, if the Black newborn babies were cared for by Black physicians, the disparity was reduced to 173 more deaths per 100,000 births compared to White newborn babies, a 58% reduction in deaths. The difference in death rates was more pronounced if the babies were sicker. Furthermore, the effects were more pronounced at hospitals where more Black babies were delivered. This difference occurred despite the fact that Black physicians were more likely to take care of more economically disadvantaged patients, take care of sicker babies, were responsible for more patients (83 versus 67 per year), and had similar levels of board certification as their White physician colleagues. Black physicians were more likely to be female. There was no difference in the mortality rate for White newborns whether they were cared for by Black physicians or White physicians. Sadly, even if White physicians had more experience taking care of Black babies, they still did not get better at saving them.

The study did offer a kernel of hope: it found that if either the Black or White physician had more formal training, the death rate for the babies decreased; and while there was still a disparity in the death rates for the Black babies cared for by White versus Black physicians, it was reduced.

This study led me to the following conclusions. Since the research study did not report any differences in the qualifications of the Black and White physicians, the only explanation I have is bias, whether implicit or explicit. Bias and racism affect babies at every level. They affect them through the negative effects on their mothers, they affect them through epigenetic changes, they even affect how much their White doctor will fight to keep them alive. If that is not a problem for America, nothing is.

Increased efforts need to be made to ensure that physicians deliver unbiased and equitable care to all their patients. In the five years I was affiliated with St. Agnes Hospital in Baltimore, each year we were required to participate in a program called TeamSTEPPS®. It is a teamwork system designed to improve communication between team members in an effort to improve the quality and safety of patient care.[6] A literature review, conducted to evaluate the program, concluded that, while further research was needed, the available research suggested that the program improved communication, reduced clinical errors, and improved patient satisfaction.[7] Effective programs in this style could be implemented to help healthcare workers reduce negative biases in delivering patient care. Program efficacy can be evaluated by monitoring changes in patient outcomes before and after implementation of training.

It should go without saying, but I will say it anyway: the physician and healthcare workforce needs to match the population. Increasing efforts should be made to increase the percentage of Black physicians from the current 5% of all physicians being Black to approximately 13%

which represents the percentage of the population in the US who are Black.

I knew I wanted to be a doctor since elementary school. More exposure of Black children to Black physicians from those early years and onward could encourage more of them to pursue medicine in the future.

The Black–White disparity in the mortality rate for Black babies is the greatest in the first seven days of the baby's life (5.71 versus 2.39),[8] but the disparity does not go away when the babies go home. In 2018 the number one cause of death among Black babies was low birthweight.[9] NH Black babies were four times as likely to die from complications of low birthweight as White babies. The number three cause was maternal complications: Black babies were 3.4 times as likely to die from maternal complications as White babies. Frankly, if we take better care of Black pregnant women, we will save more babies. I have already suggested measures to decrease the rates of low birthweight in chapter 9 and complications for Black mothers throughout the book.

Are there other opportunities for improvement? Yes. The fourth and fifth leading causes of death were sudden infant death syndrome (SIDS) and accidental injuries. Black babies were twice as likely to die for these reasons as White babies. For the second leading cause of death, congenital malformations, the Black–White disparity was lower: 1.4 to 1.

In medical school, we rotate through a number of specialties. Prior to entering medical school, my initial desire was to be a pediatrician; I was particularly diligent on that rotation. I remember an experienced female physician citing this phrase to reduce SIDS, "Not on my tum, mum." I thought it was catchy and easy to remember. The "Back to Sleep" campaign, which was initiated in 1994, reduced the rates of SIDS by 50%.[10]

The campaign did not appear to be as effective in Black communities. Black babies are less likely to be put to sleep on their backs and more than 3.5 times as likely to share a bed as White babies.[11] Bed-sharing has also been associated with an increased risk of SIDS for Black babies, twice the risk compared to Black babies who did not bed share, according to a small Chicago study.[12] The study matched 260 (case) babies, who died from SIDS, to controls. The controls were babies who were matched on specific criteria to ensure they were otherwise similar to the case babies. There are some factors that made SIDS more likely to occur when mothers share their beds with their babies, included if the mother smoked, if the baby was younger (less than one month), if pillows were used and the sleep surface was soft. It is notable that they did not find an increased risk of SIDS among bed-sharing babies whose mothers were nonsmokers, bed-sharing babies whose mothers did not smoke in pregnancy, and babies older than one month. Additionally, the authors found that breastfeeding and allowing the baby to use a pacifier were protective against SIDS.

A separate study, which looked into reasons that African American women in Washington, DC, and Maryland, gave for the choice of sleeping arrangement, should give us pause.[13] While this study again had only a small number of women (73), the subjects included women of both upper and lower socioeconomic status. Sixty percent of the babies slept with their parents at least part of the night, and more than 95% slept in the same room as their parents. The major decision factors for bed-sharing were "space/availability, convenience and safety," and comfort. Some mothers did not have space for a crib or resources to afford a crib for their babies. Some mothers found it more convenient to share a bed in that it allowed for breast and formula feeding and for recovery, "especially after cesarean sections." Some mothers thought that the babies slept better in their beds and that babies "did not like the crib." Finally, one of the primary reasons for parents' decision was safety: some mothers shared beds with their babies because they thought they could monitor their babies more closely due to concerns about their babies dying in the crib. For mothers of low socioeconomic status additional safety concerns included protecting the babies from random kidnapping, stray gunfire, and insects and other pests. It's not that they did not know that bed-sharing had risks, but they thought their choice was the safer option.

I remember the bed-sharing dilemma I faced with my own children. I was aware of the literature and the recommended precautions. For my son, it worked well. My husband dutifully brought him to our bed to breastfeed and returned him to his crib in the close by room. For my daughter, it was not that easy. Her brother had the only room that was close by, so we kept her crib next to our bed. I was able to reach over for her to breastfeed, but for whatever reason our daughter refused to fall asleep in the crib. Conflicted but exhausted, I sometimes gave up. She won. In and out of sleep I tried my best to guard her from any risk of accidental injury or other harm associated with bed-sharing. Thankfully, she remained safe.

The studies give us important information about counseling Black patients. It is still important to inform them of the known risks of bed-sharing and SIDS. It is also equally important to inform them of the factors that can reduce their risk, such as pacifier use and breastfeeding, or increase their risk such as smoking. Last but by no means least, allow our patients to share their barriers. If any barriers can be eliminated, we should direct the patients to the resources to do so. If not, we need to display empathy, even if we disagree with their decision.

The heightened fear that Black mothers may have about the life of their children is justified. That same concern may act as a barrier to recommended safe sleeping, something that can reduce SIDS and accidental injuries in bed.[14] But it is still not the main reason why more Black babies die in their first year of life. The responsibility still falls on our society in America and our failure to adequately invest in the health and well-being of our Black mothers. It falls on failures of physicians and other healthcare professionals to recognize that they are not doing as much as they could to save the lives of Black babies, as they do for White babies.

Maybe we need to take a cue from the movies. As I mentioned I love movies. I am also a fan of John Grisham. Years ago, I watched the movie *A Time to Kill*. Matthew McConaughey played a lawyer who defended a father, played by Samuel Jackson, who shot and killed two men who viciously attacked his ten-year-old daughter. In his closing argument, the lawyer asked the courtroom to close their eyes. He slowly described the horrific details of how the little girl was tied, raped, urinated on, beaten, hung, and left her for dead. He concluded: "I want you to picture the little girl. Now, imagine she's White."[15]

The Ray of Hope

I am a sucker for a happy ending. I make deliberate choices when selecting the movies I watch and the books I read. But, for far too many Black women in America, their pregnancy story does not have a happy ending. Things don't just "work out." Concerns are dismissed. Care is delayed or even denied until it is too late. Then the "if only" begins. People make excuses. They blame, sometimes appropriately, sometimes less so.

I think of a painful parallel: mass killings in schools. I think of the police or security being blamed for not acting quickly or timely enough. It's not that they couldn't have or shouldn't have acted differently, but their failure should not be used to deflect from the bigger problem, namely allowing adolescents to have weapons of war without military training or need on domestic streets.

The morbidity and mortality rates for Black women will improve if their health needs are addressed before they get pregnant. They will do better if they receive compassionate and medically sound prenatal care. They will do better if their concerns are addressed appropriately as soon as they are raised—not hours or days or weeks later. Because, even if heroic actions save some in the end, they won't save all who could have been saved if the right measures had been put in place sooner.

There has been a start. The "Preventing Maternal Death Acts of 2018" became law on December 21, 2018. In an effort to help states improve maternal health and to eliminate health disparities in "pregnancy-related and pregnancy-associated deaths,"[1] the CDC was authorized to increase state and tribal funding for maternal mortality review committees (MMRCs).[2] If it were not for those types of committees, as I discussed in chapter 7, we would not have known that over 60% of the deaths are preventable and continued and worsening disproportionate negative impact of the maternal mortality crisis on Black women.

Other legislation appears to be on its way. The Maternal Health Quality Improvement Act, will provide funding to support access to maternal care in rural communities, training to reduce and prevent discrimination in the delivery of maternal healthcare, and funding for programs that improve the quality of perinatal care delivered.[3]

The Black Maternal Health Momnibus Act of 2021 goes further. Representative Lauren Underwood, who introduced the bill,[4] was a personal friend of Dr. Shalon Irving. This bill is particularly important on many levels. It addresses multiple reasons for the disparities in Black maternal health and the maternal health disparities of other at-risk communities. If enacted, and if the resources allocated are used effectively, I believe this bill could really help to turn the tide and improve Black maternal health in this country. If the bill is passed, among other initiatives, investments will be made in housing, transportation, and nutrition to support women in the perinatal period. The community organizations, which have been working hard to support maternal health and improve equity, will receive funding. Investments will be made to expand and diversify the workforce that cares for mothers in the perinatal period to ensure that every mother receives the culturally competent care they need. Maternal mental health will be supported. Data collection processes and quality measures will be improved to allow continued understanding of the causes and the solutions.[5] Investments will be made in digital tools to improve maternal outcomes in underserved areas. Innovative payment models will be promoted "to incentivize high-quality maternity care and non-clinical perinatal support." Throughout this book, I have discussed evidence to support the need for such funding and suggestions on how resources could be allocated.

In December 2021, Vice President Kamala Harris announced a call to action to improve the health of parents and children in the first federal Maternal Health Day of Action.[6] A number of private entities detailed ways in which they planned to support maternal health. Several public sector investments were also described. Notable among the public sector initiatives is a call for states to expand Medicaid postpartum coverage to 12 months.[7] Studies have shown that in states with Medicaid expansion, uninsured rates are lower and Medicaid coverage rates are higher.[8] As we are sometimes painfully aware, it takes time for legislation to be approved, and in the interim the lives of more Black mothers will be at stake. Large organizations mean well, but depending on their size, implementation takes time. Fortunately, smaller community organizations, many whose advocacy has led to these initiatives, are still working to ensure that progress is made.

Dr. Wanda Irving and partners have set up Dr. Shalon's Maternal Action Project to continue to honor the life and legacy of her daughter Shalon.

"I see inequity wherever it exists. I am not afraid to call it by name and work hard to eliminate it. I vow to create a better earth," are the words of Shalon Irving.[9]

Recognizing that Black pregnant women need increased community support, they have created the BelieveHer App as a means of providing some of that much needed support. The ultimate goal of the app is to assist women in obtaining support from peer counselors including doulas to provide guidance on their birth journey. Women are able to receive this support while remaining anonymous.[10]

Wanda Irving's work is not easy. It takes a personal toll each time she shares her daughter's story. There is always an empty chair at her dinner table during Christmas and Thanksgiving: Shalon's chair. Wanda Irving has to explain to Shalon's daughter, Soleil, why her mommy can't come home. Yet, despite everything, she maintains hope and continues to strive to make it better for other mothers, other families.

I first heard Dr. Joia Crear-Perry speak in June 2017. It was at a meeting on Capitol Hill highlighting the issues of maternal health. The meeting was organized by ACOG under the leadership of Dr. Haywood Brown, the College's sixty-eighth president, a Maternal and Fetal Medicine specialist, who has held multiple leadership positions and has been committed to caring for women at risk for adverse pregnancy outcomes, particularly disadvantaged women, and addressing health disparities.[11] Dr. Crear-Perry spoke passionately on the issue of Black maternal health. Through her organization, the National Birth Equity Collaborative, she continues to advocate for improvement in Black maternal and infant health. In addition, her team is involved with research, education, and training.[12] Recognizing the importance of doulas for Black maternal health, her organization endorses the Birthmark Doula Collective. I met Dr. Crear-Perry in person in April 2019, when I had the pleasure to be on a panel to discuss Black maternal health. The event was a watch party, held in collaboration with the March of Dimes, and the panel was led by the March of Dimes president and CEO, Stacey D. Stewart. We were viewing an episode of the television show, *The Resident*, which was based on the true story of Kira Johnson in the hours before her death.[13] Dr. Crear-Perry was even more engaging up close and personal; she was warm and personable. She not only "talked the talk," but she also "walked the walk."

I remember another group who was present at that June 2017 event on Capitol Hill. It was the Black Mammas Matter Alliance—an alliance led by Black women working to improve the health of Black women and birthing people through enhancements and innovations in Black maternal care and research.[14] In addition, they aim to advocate for and advance policy change and shift the existing culture as it relates to Black maternal health. Among other initiatives, the alliance launched the "Black Maternal Health Week" campaign, which was officially recognized by the White House in April 2021 and which takes place every year from April 11 to 17.[15]

Emily Little has a PhD in experimental psychology. In 2017, she founded Nuturely, an organization dedicated to improving the wellness of parents and infants in the perinatal period.[16] Little's international work exposed her to the importance of community in the perinatal period, something she found deficient in the United States. Her organization is committed to equity and recognizes the barriers placed by "racism and systemic oppression."

Sabia Wade is the President of the Board of Nuturely. She is a doula, speaker, coach, and entrepreneur who is committed to improving inclusion, diversity, and equity in reproductive justice and other domains.[17] Our paths crossed when I was invited to participate in a conference on "Racism in Perinatal and Pediatric Health," a 6-week virtual workshop for Oregon health professionals held in early 2021. The aim was to provide education and guidance to these professionals to help them deliver more equitable, culturally sensitive care. Both Emily Little and Sabia Wade, the workshop organizers, have impressed me with their drive, with their commitment to, and their passion for, the work of improving the health and wellness of Black women in the perinatal period and of other groups who suffer from racism and other barriers to competent and compassionate care.

Among the speakers at the workshop was one I had heard before. His name is Dr. Neel Shah, an Assistant Professor at Harvard Medical School. I had heard Dr. Shah present at grand rounds early in my time at Yale. Since we were in the first year of the pandemic, 2020, the presentation was virtual. I knew nothing about him before I heard him speak at Yale, but his presentation, which discussed the importance of a cohesive and communicative delivery team in the care of mothers in the obstetric unit, impressed me. When I learned more about all the work he had done in maternal health, I was even more impressed. In his current role as Chief Medical Officer at Maven Clinic he continues to strongly advocate for and innovate programs to support Black mothers in the perinatal period.[18]

Another vocal advocate for Black maternal health is SciHonor Devotion, whom I wrote about in chapter 10. She not only continues her work in educating doulas and supporting Black mothers, but has pursued further studies in midwifery. In addition to other services, her organization, Earth's Natural Touch Birth Care and Beyond, offers a weekly virtual breastfeeding support group, Mocha Milkshake Café.[19]

The efficacy of initiatives must be evaluated. Proven interventions need to be implemented, and their outcomes—in terms of tangible changes in Black maternal health and infant outcome—need to be measured to ensure that the implementation at least reaches the standard of the initial initiative. New innovations need to be developed and successful ones adopted.

While leading two health centers for the Baltimore Medical System, I had to learn and implement PDSAs (Plan, Do, Study, Act), brief cycles of interventions with specific measurable goals.[20] The outcome was documented, and lessons were learned whether the intervention was successful or not. The hope was that successful interventions would be implemented on a larger scale. Even in our low-resource setting, we were able to plan, do, and study multiple such initiatives. Nevertheless, resources, especially human capital, are needed to support full-scale implementation of successful initiatives. I often found the champions of the work to be physicians who were passionate about the care they were delivering to patients. However, due to clinical duties their time was limited. They were ably supported by medical assistants, who were equally passionate about the care, but who also found it difficult to divide their time between the initiatives due to their other clinical responsibilities.

Sometimes the projects were effective, but due to changes in the workforce they often could not be sustained. However, I still was able to see the potential of these projects. Working with these physician-champions reinforced and enhanced the lessons I had learned about physicians who still choose to deliver mainly clinical care. They have innovative ideas based on their experience and, if given the support, including financial, technical, and human capital, some are capable of implementing improvements that extend far beyond the individual interaction in the exam room. Many do not want to leave patient care; they just need a little time and space to grow beyond that role—an opportunity they are seldom given, due to obligations of seeing multiple patients in a short span of time.

While we recognize that our physician workforce needs to develop its delivery of culturally sensitive care, let's not forget that the workforce consists of human beings. Human beings who often have altruist reasons to pursue medicine, to pursue obstetric care, but imperfect human beings, nonetheless. If these human beings are overly burdened like many are now, if the demands on them continue to grow, many may be led to decrease the hours they devote to the field of obstetrics or other fields of medicine, or leave the field completely. For many, the toll could be even worse. The suicide rate among male physicians is 40% higher than the general suicide rate for men, and among female physicians that number is 130% higher.[21] According to a Medscape 2021 survey, on average, 13% of physicians have had suicidal thoughts. For OB/GYNs it is even worse: they topped with list with 19% reporting suicidal thoughts.[22] Let's not forget that, as a country, America will likely continue its trend of worsening maternal health for women, and even more so Black women, if the caregivers, the physicians, and other health professionals are not cared for. These clinicians need to be allocated sufficient time and resources to continue in their vocation of caring for women.

As investment continues for the care of Black mothers, responsible, passionate, goal-oriented champions need to be identified and nurtured, so they can plan new initiatives and advance care. Some initiatives need to be on a scale small enough to be carried out in the short term. If successful, they should be quickly implemented and if not, they should be abandoned with the lessons learned carefully documented. We cannot solely rely on long-term solutions. In addition to measures in maternal-health outcomes for Black women and their babies, it is equally important to measure whether healthcare professionals and institutions have improved their delivery of care to Black patients in a culturally sensitive and unbiased manner.

One of the difficulties has been how to measure this outcome. How do we measure the racism that Black women experience while receiving their obstetric care? Dr. Karen Scott, whom I have never met, recognizes this need. She is an obstetrician and gynecologist with an MPH from Emory University and founder and CEO of Birthing Cultural Rigor, LLC.[23] She developed and, with a large team of other researchers, validated the Patient Reported Experience Measure of OBstetric racism©, also known as the PREM-OB Scale™.[24] The tool was rigorously developed building on previously devised standards through a collaboration between individuals, including "Black women scholars, Black women-led community organizations, non-Black health services researchers, and Black mothers and birthing people."[25] The tool offers a means to quantitatively measure the experiences of Black mothers and birthing people in the hospital in order to "quantify obstetric racism for use in perinatal improvement initiatives."[26]

I have highlighted only a few of the great many entities and individuals that are doing the work to improve Black maternal health. There are others, and I believe all are needed and all are important. I have discussed only some solutions.

Change takes time, but it is possible. I think collaborations are key. I think large healthcare organizations and insurance companies need to continue to actively engage in the conversations and implement solutions. Medical schools and other training programs for healthcare professionals need to double down on their commitment to train knowledgeable, compassionate, and culturally competent healthcare professionals for the workforce of the future. These burgeoning health-care professionals need their humanity to be recognized so that they can receive support in developing their strengths and overcoming their weaknesses. Political leaders need to continue to work together to pass much needed legislation. Employers should be more supportive of their pregnant and postpartum patients and spare them the judgment that is generously heaped on many, often more so if they happen to be Black. Individuals can show support even if that support is only the ability to offer a kind work to a pregnant person.

Community organizations need to continue to share best prac-tices to improve the health of Black women, including pre-conception, during pregnancy, and post-delivery.

My aim in writing this book is to help to provide more information and tools to advance the work. In 2018 when I did my TEDx talk I shared the hope I had to America—hope to eliminate health disparities in maternal health and improve the maternal health for all women in America.[27] My hope is to help ensure that Shalon Irving, or any mother who died in the pregnancy and childbirth period, did not die in vain. I realize the journey is long. The journey is costly, and the journey can be painful. But as I said, I am a sucker for happy endings. I believe America has all it needs to improve Black maternal health and to elim-inate disparities. I believe that the lessons learned will improve the maternal health of all women in America. The only question I have for you is: "Are you on board?"

Acknowledgments

As I consider the journey that was completing this book, I realize it began long before I put pen to paper. Reflecting on the journey has allowed me to recognize the important role certain individuals play in my life, although I didn't always recognize the importance of their support in the moment, I would like to take the time to thank them.

That being said, I would like to start at the beginning, my parents Milton and Kathleen Rainford. You not only instilled in me the importance of education but more importantly, using the gifts that one has been blessed with to serve others. There aren't enough words to express my gratitude for the unmeasurable support you have provided me well beyond the years that it would be considered an obligation. You were my first editors, a role you continued even in many of my professional writing roles. To my Dad, thank you for sharing your vision that I should write another "pregnancy book" and my mother for your confidence that I could accomplish the goal even when I felt the odds were against me. I am so grateful that I am blessed with you both as parents and I love you always.

To Dr. Alvin Poussaint, the former Associate Dean for Student Affairs at Harvard Medical School and the founding Director of the Office of Recruitment & Multicultural Affairs. Your role and presence were key in helping to make Harvard Medical School the welcoming environment I felt it to be so many years ago. I still recall the honor I felt when you welcomed us as students into your home. I may not have realized the significance at the time, but I definitely felt the love and support. Thank you for all you have done.

To Dr. Anthony Scialli, the Residency Program Director in the Department of Obstetrics and Gynecology, during my time at Georgetown. Your somewhat unconventional style encouraged me to challenge the status quo. Thank you for sharing your wisdom and encouraging me to think outside of the box.

To the American College of Obstetricians and Gynecologists. I have relied on the valuable and regularly updated information you have provided over the years to keep me up-to-date in the specialty and to help to ensure I was providing my patients with the high standard of care they deserved. The pomp and ceremony of being inducted as a Fellow provided a special moment that I was able to share with my parents. Your weekday newsletter "ACOG Today's Headlines" exposed me to the articles that expanded my understanding of the disparities that exist for black women in America. Thank you for continuing to strive to improve your service to women's health.

Nina Martin, you are a journalist extraordinaire. Thank you for your outstanding service to women's health, especially your "Lost Mothers" project. Your in depth, well-researched and very deeply personal stories of mothers who have lost their lives in the perinatal period helped to ignite my passion to do more. Thank you for accepting an email from me, a perfect stranger at the time, and connecting me with Mrs. Wanda Irving.

Linda Villarosa as a journalist, author and educator par excellence, not only did your work inspire me on this journey of trying to address maternal health disparities, but you also selflessly assisted me in determining the best direction for this book. Thank you for your kindness and your generosity. It is a gift to know you.

To Dr. Amy Holda Gueye-Weinstein for sharing your entrepreneurial ideas which re-sparked my interest in writing about pregnancy. Thank you for starting this journey with me and recognizing when it was time for me to continue on the road alone.

I would like to thank my agent and friend Sha-Shana Crichton. Thank you for believing in me and knowing that I could fulfill this important role and staying the course on this multiyear journey. Thank you for your patience in allowing me to recognize the book that I needed to write rather than the book I thought I wanted to write. I am fortunate that I can count you as one of my dearest friends.

I would like to thank Donna Hemans for your professional role in editing my book proposals. Thank you for your availability and guidance.

To my classmate from Harvard Medical School, Dr. Neal Baer. Thank you for taking the time to allow me to share this idea with you and for introducing me to Linda, who was just the person I needed to shape the vision of this book to the one that needed to be written. I will forever be impressed that you were my classmate who wrote for the hit television series ER. I am continually impressed by all the work that you have done.

I would like to thank Dr. David Katz, for your willingness to offer me thoughtful advice on multiple occasions and for endorsing the importance of this book at a time when I was uncertain as to whether I should proceed on my quest to bring it to reality.

Adrienne Ingrum, thank you for remembering me and giving me the opportunity to pitch to Broadleaf Books. I feel honored that you gave me this chance. Without you this book may never have come to fruition.

Thank you to Lisa Kloskin and Jarrod Harrison. I appreciated your excellent guidance and editorial support. I am grateful to be part of a team that I know has my back. It has been a joy to work with you both.

To the production editor, Rachel Reyes, for your attention to detail to ensure that my words had their intended meaning.

To Mrs. Wanda Irving, thank you for allowing me to share the story of your dear daughter Dr. Shalon Irving even before we had ever met. Thank you for allowing me to continue to be a part of your life and giving me insight into your journey of effecting change. You are an incredible person, and I am grateful to know you.

I would like to thank Dr. Lanetta Bronté-Hall, Dr. Megan Clowse and Dr. Oneeka Willams, incredible physician leaders. Thank you for sharing your stories with me and thank you for all you continue to do to make change.

Claudia Ferguson's mother, Ms. Colatha Bolt, thank you for allowing me to share your daughter's story in this way. Claudia inspired me to do more for sickle cell disease and I am glad I can play a small role in continuing her legacy.

To Emma White, Bethany Stone, Ariel Banks and Dr. Sally Ward, you know who you are, thank you for bravely sharing your stories with me and allowing me to bring a personal element to the experiences of black women. Each of you is an outstanding individual who is charting a course to make this world a better place.

I would like to thank all the researchers. Your often unsung efforts have allowed us to gain a quantitative understanding of the negative effects of the current healthcare system on the health of black women and the exciting opportunities for us to do better.

I would like to thank all the advocacy groups in the black maternal health space including Dr. Joia Crear-Perry the founder and president of the National Birth Equity Collaborative and the Black Mamas Matter Alliance. Thank you for continually highlighting the inequities and to advocate and insist that the lives of black mothers need to be valued.

I would like to thank two of my closest friends, Dr. Jacqueline Duncan and Dr. Andrea Isaacs. You are phenomenal women who continue to do great things. You have continued to stand by me in my highs and lows and your support in this process has been priceless.

To my dear brothers, Norman and Ryan. It is beyond good fortune to have brothers like you. You both have proven multiple times that I can always count on you. Your role and presence in my life define the term in the best possible light.

To the three loves of my life, my children, Zane and Kia, thank you for being patient even when it looks like your mother is always at her desk. Thank you for your love and laughter. I value your insatiable curiosity and your strong opinions even if at times I may tell you otherwise. You are my greatest joy! And my husband Ryan, thank you for being my biggest supporter, my best friend and my life partner, and the answer to a prayer.

To God be the glory!

Notes

Prelude

1 Kiranpreet Kaur, Mamta Bhardwaj, Prasant Kumar, Suresh Singhal, Taran-deep Singh, and Sarla Hooda, "Amniotic Fluid Embolism, *Journal of Anaes-thesiology Clinical Pharmacology* 32, no. 2 (April–June 2016): 153–159. https://www.ncbi.nlm.nih.gov/pmc/articles/PMC4874066/.

Introduction

1 https://www.propublica.org/article/lost-mothers-maternal-health-died-childbirth-pregnancy
2 https://www.ted.com/talks/miriam_zoila_perez_how_racism_harms_pregnant_women_and_what_can_help?language=en
3 https://www.ted.com/talks/david_r_williams_how_racism_makes_us_sick?language=en
4 Monique Rainford, "America's Maternal Nightmare," Filmed September 27, 2018, TED video, https://www.ted.com/talks/monique_rainford_america_s_maternal_nightmare.

Chapter 1

1 Zinzi D. Bailey et al., "Structural Racism and Health Inequities in the USA," *Lancet* 389, no. 10077 (April 2017): 1453–1463. https://doi.org/10.1016/S0140-6736(17)30569-X; Nancy Kreiger, "Discrimination and Health Inequities," *International Journal of Health Services* 44, no. 4 (2014): 643–710. https://doi.org/0.2190/HS.44.4.b.
2 David R. Roediger, "Historical Foundations of Race," National Museum of African American History and Culture, accessed April 17, 2022, https://nmaahc.si.edu/learn/talking-about-race/topics/historical-foundations-race.

3 Mike Cummings, "Numbers, Not Narratives, Remedy Misperceptions of the Racial Wealth Gap," Yale News, September 13, 2021, https://news.yale.edu/2021/09/13/numbers-not-narratives-remedy-misperceptions-racial-wealth-gap.

4 #lifestylemed2018, Twitter, last accessed April 17, 2022. https://twitter.com/hashtag/lifestylemed2018?src=hash.

5 "What is Epigenetics?," Center for Disease Control and Prevention, last updated May 18, 2022, https://www.cdc.gov/genomics/disease/epigenetics.htm.

6 Lawrence Wallack and Kent Thornburg, "Developmental Origins, Epigenetics, and Equity: Moving Upstream," Maternal Child Health Journal 20, no. 5 (May 2016): 935–940. https://doi.org/10.1007/s10995-016-1970-8.

7 Kent L. Thornburg et al., "In Utero Life and Epigenetic Predisposition for Disease," Advances in Genetics, no. 71 (2010): 57–78. https://doi.org/10.1016/B978-0-12-380864-6.00003-1.

8 https://www.npr.org/sections/codeswitch/2018/01/14/577664626/making-the-case-that-discrimination-is-bad-for-your-health

9 Arline T. Geronimus et al., "'Weathering' and Age Patterns of Allostatic Load Scores Among Blacks and Whites in the United States," American Journal of Public Health 96, no. 5 (May 2006): 826–833. https://doi.org/10.2105/AJPH.2004.060749.

10 B.S. McEwen and E. Stellar, "Stress and the Individual: Mechanisms Leading to Disease," Archives of Internal Medicine 153, no. 18 (September 1993): 2093–2101. https://doi.org/10.1001/archinte.1993.00410180039004.

11 Geronimus et al., "'Weathering' and Age Patterns."

12 Teresa E. Seeman et al., "Allostatic Load as a Marker of Cumulative Biological Risk: MacArthur Studies of Successful Aging," PNAS 98, no. 8 (April 2001): 4770–4775. https://doi.org/10.1073/pnas.081072698.

13 J. Guidi et al., "Allostatic Load and Its Impact on Health: A Systematic Review," Psychotherapy and Psychosomatics 90, no. 11 (2021): 11–27. https://doi.org/10.1159/000510696.

14 Masood A. Shammas, "Telomeres, Lifestyle, Cancer, and Aging," Current Opinion in Clinical Nutrition & Metabolic Care 14, no. 1 (January 2011): 28–34. https://doi.org/10.1097/MCO.0b013e32834121b1.

15 Arline T. Geronimus et al., "Do US Black Women Experience Stress-Related Accelerated Biological Aging? A Novel Theory and First Population-Based Test of Black–White Differences in Telomere Length," Human Nature 21, no. 1 (March 2010): 19–38. https://doi.org/10.1007/s12110-010-9078-0.

16 Karen Hughes et al., "The Effect of Multiple Adverse Childhood Experiences on Health: A Systematic Review and Meta-analysis," Lancet Public Health 2, no. 8 (2017): e356–366. https://doi.org/10.1016/S2468-2667(17)30118-4.

17 Vanessa Sacks and David Murphey, "The Prevalence of Adverse Childhood Experiences, Nationally, by State, and by Race or Ethnicity," Child Trends, February 12, 2018, https://www.childtrends.org/publications/prevalence-adverse-childhood-experiences-nationally-state-race-ethnicity.

18 New York City Department of Health and Mental Hygiene, "Severe Maternal Morbidity: New York City, 2008–2012," City of New York, 2016, https://www1.

nyc.gov/assets/doh/downloads/pdf/data/maternal-morbidity-report-08-12.
pdf.

19 Chloë FitzGerald and Samia Hurst, "Implicit Bias in Healthcare Professionals: A Systematic Review," *BMC Medical Ethics*, no. 18 (2017): art. 19. https://doi.org/10.1186/s12910-017-0179-8.

20 Alexander R. Green et al., "Implicit Bias among Physicians and its Prediction of Thrombolysis Decisions for Black and White Patients," *Journal of General Internal Medicine* 22, no. 9 (2007): 1231–1238. https://doi.org/10.1007/s11606-007-0258-5; Elizabeth N. Chapman, Anna Kaatz, and Molly Carnes, "Physicians and Implicit Bias: How Doctors May Unwittingly Perpetuate Health Care Disparities," *Journal of General Internal Medicine* 28, no. 11 (November 2013): 1504–1510. https://doi.org/10.1007/s11606-013-2441-1.

21 Janice A. Sabin, Brian A. Nosek, Anthony G. Greenwald, and Frederick P. Rivara, "Physicians' Implicit and Explicit Attitudes About Race by MD Race, Ethnicity, and Gender," *Journal of Health Care for the Poor and Underserved* 20, no. 3 (August 2009): 896–913. https://doi.org/10.1353/hpu.0.0185.

22 Bentley L. Gibson et al., "Sources of Implicit and Explicit Intergroup Race Bias among African-American Children and Young Adults," *PloS One* 12, no. 9 (September 2017): e0183015. https://doi.org/10.1371/journal.pone.0183015.

23 Patricia G. Devine, Patrick S. Forscher, Anthony J. Austin, and William T. L. Cox, "Long-Term Reduction in Implicit Race Bias: A Prejudice Habit-Breaking Intervention," *Journal of Experimental Social Psychology* 48, no. 6 (November 2012): 1267–1278. https://doi.org/10.1016/j.jesp.2012.06.003.

Chapter 2

1 "Infertility FAQs, " Center for Disease Control and Prevention, last updated March 1, 2022, https://www.cdc.gov/reproductivehealth/infertility/index.htm.

2 Elizabeth Hervey Stephen and Anjani Chandra, "Declining Estimates of Infertility in the United States: 1982–2002," *Fertility and Sterility* 86, no. 3 (2006): 516–523. https://doi.org/10.1016/j.fertnstert.2006.02.129.

3 Melissa F. Wellons et al., "Racial Differences in Self-Reported Infertility and Risk Factors for Infertility in a Cohort of Black and White Women: The CARDIA Women's Study," *Fertility and Sterility* 90, no. 5 (2008): 1640–1648. https://doi.org/10.1016/j.fertnstert.2007.09.056.

4 Roxane C. Handal-Orefice, Melissa McHale, Alexander M. Friedman, Joseph A. Politch, and Wendy Kuohung, "Impact of Race Versus Ethnicity on Infertility Diagnosis Between Black American, Haitian, African, and White American Women Seeking Infertility Care: A Retrospective Review," *F&S Reports* 3, no. 2 Suppl. (May 2022): 22–28. https://doi.org/10.1016/j.xfre.2021.11.003.

5 Alexandra Minna Stern, "That Time the United States Sterilized 60,000 of Its Citizens," *Huffpost*, January 7, 2016, https://www.huffpost.com/entry/sterilization-united-states_n_568f35f2e4b0c8beacf68713.

6 Alexandra Minna Stern, "Forced Sterilization Policies in the US Targeted Minorities and Those with Disabilities—and Lasted Into the 21st Century," University of Michigan Institute for Healthcare and Policy and Innovation

News, September 23, 2020, https://ihpi.umich.edu/news/forced-sterilization-policies-us-targeted-minorities-and-those-disabilities-and-lasted-21st.

7   Erica Cohn, dir. *Belly of the Beast* (Belly of the Beast LLC, Idle Wild Films, Independent Television Services & Black Public Media, 2020).

8   Julia Naftulin, "Inside the Hidden Campaign to Forcibly Steril-ize Thousands of Inmates in California Women's Prisons," *Insider*, November 24, 2020, https://www.insider.com/inside-forced-sterilizations-california-womens-prisons-documentary-2020-11.

9   Thomas W. Volscho, "Sterilization Racism and Pan-ethnic Disparities of the Last Decade: The Continued Encroachment on Reproductive Rights," *Wicazo Sa Review: A Journal of Native American Studies*, 25, no. 1 (2010): 17–31. https://doi.org/10.1353/wic.0.0053.

10 Sonya B. Borrero et al., "Race, Insurance Status, and Desire for Tubal Ster-ilization Reversal," *Fertil Steril* 90, no. 2 (August 2008): 272–277. https://doi.org/10.1016/j.fertnstert.2007.06.041.

11 Richard Gawel, "Hispanic, Black Women Less Likely to Use Fertility Treat-ment Even with Insurance Coverage," Women's Health & OB/GYN, October 18, 2021, https://www.healio.com/news/womens-health-ob-gyn/20211018/hispanic-black-women-less-likely-to-use-fertility-treatment-even-with-insurance-coverage.

12 Jamie Blynn, "Gabrielle Union on Infertility, Surrogacy: 'Every Route to Par-enthood is Perfect,'" Today, January 23, 2019, https://www.today.com/parents/gabrielle-union-infertility-surrogacy-new-baby-girl-t147325.

13 Usha Lee McFarling, "For Black Women, the Isolation of Infertility is Compounded by Barriers to Treatment," Stat, October 14, 2020, https://www.statnews.com/2020/10/14/for-black-women-isolation-of-infertility-compounded-by-barriers-to-treatment/.

14 Elizabeth Grow, "'How Dare You Adopt a White Baby?!' 'We Only Had the Desire to Become Parents': Couple Battling Male Factor Infertility Build Tran-sracial Family through Adoption, Embryo Donations," Love What Matters, accessed June 11, 2022, https://www.lovewhatmatters.com/couple-battling-male-factor-infertility-build-transracial-family-through-adoption-embryo-donations/.

15 Amy Dockser Marcus, "Sperm Banks Struggle to Recruit Black Donors and Other Donors of Color," *Wall Street Journal*, February 26, 2022, https://www.wsj.com/articles/sperm-banks-struggle-to-recruit-black-donors-and-other-donors-of-color-11645887602.

Chapter 3

1   Carla Dugas and Valori H. Slane, "Miscarriage," National Library of Medicine, last updated May 8, 2022, https://www.ncbi.nlm.nih.gov/books/NBK532992/.

2   Siobhan Quenby et al., "Miscarriage Matters: The Epidemiological, Physical, Psychological, and Economic Costs of Early Pregnancy Loss," *Lancet* 397, no. 10285 (May 2021): 1658–1667. https://doi.org/10.1016/S0140-6736(21)00682-6.

3 Sudeshna Mukherjee et al., "Risk of Miscarriage Among Black Women and White Women in a US Prospective Cohort Study," *American Journal of Epidemiology* 177, no. 11 (June 2013): 1271–1278. https://doi.org/10.1093/aje/kws393.

4 Sarah Prager, Elizabeth Micks, and Vanessa K. Dalton, "Pregnancy Loss (Miscarriage): Terminology, Risk Factors, and Etiology," UpToDate, last updated September 24, 20021, https://www.uptodate.com/contents/pregnancy-loss-miscarriage-terminology-risk-factors-and-etiology.

5 Siobhan Quenby et al., "Miscarriage Matters: The Epidemiological, Physical, Psychological, and Economic Costs of Early Pregnancy Loss," *Lancet* 397, no. 10285 (May 2021): 1658–1667. https://doi.org/10.1016/S0140-6736(21)00682-6.

6 Rochelle S. Green, Brian Malig, Gayle C. Windham, Laura Fenster, Bart Ostro, and Shanna Swan, "Residential Exposure to Traffic and Spontaneous Abortion," *Environmental Health Perspectives* 117, no. 12 (December 2009): 1939–1944. https://doi.org/10.1289/ehp.0900943.

7 "Smoking During Pregnancy," Center for Disease Control and Prevention, last modified April 28, 2020, https://www.cdc.gov/tobacco/basic_information/health_effects/pregnancy/index.htm.

8 Christopher W. Tessum, David A. Paolella, Sarah E. Chambliss, Joshua S. Apte, Jason D. Hill, and Julian D. Marshall, "PM2.5 Polluters Disproportionately and Systemically Affect People of Color in the United States," *Science Advances* 7, no. 18 (April 2021), https://doi.org/10.1126/sciadv.abf4491.

9 Elizabeth A. Stewart et al., "The Burden of Uterine Fibroids for African-American Women: Results of a National Survey," *Journal of Womens Health* 22, no. 10 (October 2013): 807–816. https://doi.org/10.1089/jwh.2013.4334.

10 Heba M. Eltoukhi et al., "The Health Disparities of Uterine Fibroids for African American Women: A Public Health Issue," *American Journal of Obstetrics and Gynecology* 210, no. 3 (March 2014): 194. https://doi.org/10.1016/j.ajog.2013.08.008.

11 Amelia K. Wesselink et al., "A Prospective Cohort Study of Ambient Air Pollution Exposure and Risk of Uterine Leiomyomata," *Human Reproduction 36*, no. 8 (August 2021): 2321–2330. https://doi.org/10.1093/humrep/deab095.

12 Fan Qu et al., "The Association between Psychological Stress and Miscarriage: A Systematic Review and Meta-Analysis," *Scientific Reports* 7 (2017): art. 1731. https://doi.org/10.1038/s41598-017-01792-3.

13 Teresa E. Seeman et al., "Allostatic Load as a Marker of Cumulative Biological Risk: MacArthur Studies of Successful Aging," *PNAS* 98, no. 8 (April 2001): 4770–4775. https://doi.org/10.1073/pnas.081072698.

14 Qu et al., "The Association between Psychological Stress and Miscarriage," 4.

15 Lars P.A. Brandt and Claus V. Nielsen, "Job Stress and Adverse Outcome of Pregnancy: A Causal Link or Recall Bias?," *American Journal of Epidemiology* 135, no. 3 (1992): 302–311. https://doi.org/10.1093/oxfordjournals.aje.a116284.

16 Tom O'Hare and Francis Creed, "Life Events and Miscarriage," *British Journal of Psychiatry* 167, no. 6 (January 1995): 799–805. https://doi.org/10.1192/bjp.167.6.799.

17 "Black Women & the Pay Gap," American Association of University Women, accessed June 10, 2022, https://www.aauw.org/resources/article/black-women-and-the-pay-gap/.

18 Rebecca Pifer, "Black Women Disproportionately Concentrated in Low-Wage, Hazardous Healthcare Jobs, Study Finds," HealthcareDive, February 8, 2022, https://www.healthcaredive.com/news/black-women-disproportionately-concentrated-low-wage-hazardous-health-jobs/618471/.

19 Gillian B. White, "Black Workers Really Do Need to Be Twice as Good," *Atlantic*, October 7, 2015, https://www.theatlantic.com/business/archive/2015/10/why-black-workers-really-do-need-to-be-twice-as-good/409276/.

20 Susan Green, "Violence Against Black Women—Many Types, Far-Reaching Effects," Institute for Women's Policy Research, July 13, 2017, https://iwpr.org/iwpr-issues/race-ethnicity-gender-and-economy/violence-against-black-women-many-types-far-reaching-effects/.

21 "Homelessness and Racial Disparities," National Alliance to End Homelessness, updated October 2020, https://endhomelessness.org/homelessness-in-america/what-causes-homelessness/inequality/.

22 Robert Laumbach, Qingyu Meng, and Howard Kipen, "What Can Individuals Do to Reduce Personal Health Risks from Air Pollution?," *Journal of Thoracic Disease* 7, no. 1 (January 2015): 96–107. https://doi.org/10.3978/j.issn.2072-1439.2014.12.21.

Chapter 4

1 Enrique Rivero, "Proportion of Black Physicians in U.S. Has Changed Little in 120 Years, UCLA Research Finds," UCLA Newsroom, April 19, 2021, https://newsroom.ucla.edu/releases/proportion-black-physicians-little-change.

2 "Quick Facts: United States," United States Census Bureau, accessed May 30, 2022, https://www.census.gov/quickfacts/fact/table/US/LFE046220.

3 William F. Rayburn, Imam M. Xierali, Laura Castillo-Page, and Marc A. Nivet, "Racial and Ethnic Differences Between Obstetrician-Gynecologists and Other Adult Medical Specialists," *Obstetrics & Gynecology* 127, no. 1 (January 2016): 148–152. http://doi.org/10.1097/AOG.0000000000001184.

4 Judith Solomon, "Closing the Coverage Gap Would Improve Black Maternal Health," Center on Budget and Policy Priorities, July 26, 2021, https://www.cbpp.org/research/health/closing-the-coverage-gap-would-improve-black-maternal-health.

5 Hannah Nelson, "OBGYNs Face Challenges When Providing Care to Medicaid Members," Healthpayer Intelligence, March 4, 2021, https://healthpayerintelligence.com/news/obgyns-face-challenges-when-providing-care-to-medicaid-members.

6 Linda Marsa, "Labor Pains: The OB-GYN Shortage," Association of American Medical Colleges, November 15, 2018, https://www.aamc.org/news-insights/labor-pains-ob-gyn-shortage.

7 United States Department of Health and Human Services, Health Resources and Services Administration, National Center for Health Workforce Analysis, *Projections of Supply and Demand for Women's Health Service Providers: 2018–2030*, March 2021, https://bhw.hrsa.gov/sites/default/files/bureau-health-workforce/data-research/projections-supply-demand-2018-2030.pdf.

8 J. Larry Jameson and Kevin B. Mahoney, Communication from the Dean to Faculty, Students, and Staff and UPHS Leadership, "Appointment of Elizabeth A. Howell, MD, MPP, as Chair of the Department of Obstetrics and Gynecology," Perelmann School of Medicine, University of Pennsylvania, May 12, 2020, https://www.med.upenn.edu/evpdeancommunications/2020-05-12-210.html.

9 Elizabeth A. Howell, "Reducing Disparities in Severe Maternal Morbidity and Mortality," *Clinical Obstetrics and Gynecology* 61, no. 2 (June 2018): 387–399. http://doi.org/10.1097/GRF.0000000000000349.

10 Audrey F. Saftlas, Lisa M. Koonin, and Hani K. Atrash, "Racial Disparity in Pregnancy-Related Mortality Associated with Livebirth: Can Established Risk Factors Explain It?," *American Journal of Epidemiology* 152, no. 5 (September 2000): 413–419. https://doi.org/10.1093/aje/152.5.413.

11 Elizabeth Chuck, "'An Amazing First Step': Advocates Hail Congress's Maternal Mortality Prevention Bill," U.S. News, December 19, 2018, https://www.nbcnews.com/news/us-news/amazing-first-step-advocates-hail-congress-s-maternal-mortality-prevention-n948951.

12 "Kira Johnson, Cedars-Sinai Los Angeles," Consumer Watchdog, accessed May 30, 2022, https://www.consumerwatchdog.org/patient-safety/kira-johnson-cedars-sinai-los-angeles.

13 "Our Impact," 4 Kira 4 Moms, accessed May 30, 2022, https://4kira4moms.com/who-are-we/.

14 Nelson, "OBGYNs Face Challenges."

15 "Who We Are," Irth (Birth Without Bias) App, accessed June 3, 2022, https://irthapp.com/who-we-are/.

16 "About Me," Ashlee Wisdom, accessed June 4, 2022, https://www.ashleewisdom.com/about-me.

17 Kayla Hui, "How One App Is Helping Black Women Find Culturally Competent Care," very well health, January 6, 2022, https://www.verywellhealth.com/health-in-her-hue-app-5214764.

18 "About Me," Ashlee Wisdom.

Chapter 5

1 Joyce A. Martin and Michelle J.K. Osterman, "Describing the Increase in Preterm Births in the United States, 2014–2016," *NCHS Data Brief*, no. 312 (June 2018), https://www.cdc.gov/nchs/data/databriefs/db312.pdf.

2 Joyce A. Martin and Michelle J.K. Osterman, "Exploring the Decline in the Singleton Preterm Birth Rate in the United States, 2019–2022," *NCHS Data Brief*, no. 430 (January 2022), https://www.cdc.gov/nchs/data/databriefs/db430.pdf.

3   "Preterm Birth," Centers for Disease Control and Prevention, last modified November 1, 2021, https://www.cdc.gov/reproductivehealth/maternalinfanthealth/pretermbirth.htm.

4   David Rose, "A History of the March of Dimes," March of Dimes, August 26, 2010, https://www.marchofdimes.org/mission/a-history-of-the-march-of-dimes.aspx.

5   "January 3, 1938: Franklin Roosevelt Founds March of Dimes," This Day in History, History.com, last modified January 2, 2020, https://www.history.com/this-day-in-history/franklin-roosevelt-founds-march-of-dimes.

6   "Eradicating Polio," UNICEF, accessed June 11, 2022, https://www.unicef.org/immunization/polio.

7   "Who We Are," March of Dimes, accessed June 11, 2022, https://www.marchofdimes.org/mission/who-we-are.aspx.

8   "2021 March of Dimes Report Card," March of Dimes, 2021, https://www.marchofdimes.org/materials/March-of-Dimes-2021-Full-Report-Card.pdf.

9   Kenneth D. Kochanek, Jiaquan Xu, and Elizabeth Arias, "Mortality in the United States, 2019," *NCHS Data Brief*, no. 395 (December 2020), fig. 5 data table, https://www.cdc.gov/nchs/data/databriefs/db395-H.pdf.

10 "Preterm Birth," Centers for Disease Control and Prevention.

11 Hannah Echols, "UAB Hospital Delivers Record-Breaking Premature Baby," Health & Medicine, University of Alabama News, November 10, 2021, https://www.uab.edu/news/health/item/12427-uab-hospital-delivers-record-breaking-premature-baby.

12 Erin Donnelly and Stacy Jackman, "The Emotional Story Behind the World's Most Premature Baby: 'He Was Able to Show Us That He Was Bigger and Stronger Than We Expected'," Yahoo!Life, February 23, 2022, https://www.yahoo.com/lifestyle/worlds-most-premature-baby-curtis-means-172139245.html.

13 Tracy A. Manuck, "Racial and Ethnic Differences in Preterm Birth: A Complex, Multifactorial Problem," *Seminars in Perinatology* 48, no. 8 (December 2017): 511–518. https://doi.org/10.1053/j.semperi.2017.08.010.

14 Colette N. Ncube et al., "Association of Neighborhood Context with Offspring Risk of Preterm Birth and Low Birthweight: A Systematic Review and Meta-Analysis of Population-Based Studies," *Social Science & Medicine* 153 (March 2016): 156–164. https://doi.org/10.1016/j.socscimed.2016.02.014.

15 Gene A. McGrady et al., "Preterm Delivery and Low Birth Weight Among First-Born Infants of Black and White College Graduates," *American Journal of Epidemiology* 136, no. 3 (August 1992): 266–276. https://doi.org/10.1093/oxfordjournals.aje.a116492.

16 Robert L. Goldenberg et al., "Medical, Psychosocial, and Behavioral Risk Factors Do Not Explain the Increased Risk for Low Birth Weight Among Black Women," *American Journal of Obstetrics and Gynecology* 175, no. 5 (November 1996): 1317–1324. https://doi.org/10.1016/s0002-9378(96)70048-0.

17 Manuck, "Racial and Ethnic Differences in Preterm Birth."

18 Irma T. Elo, Zoua Vang, and Jennifer F. Culhane, "Variation in Birth Outcomes by Mother's Country of Birth Among Non-Hispanic Black Women in

the United States," *Maternal and Child Health Journal* 18, no. 10 (2014): 2371–2381. https://doi.org/10.1007/s10995-014-1477-0.

19 Elo, Vang, and Culhane, "Variation in Birth Outcomes," 2379.

20 Paola Scommegna, "High Premature Birth Rates Among U.S. Black Women May Reflect the Stress of Racism and Health and Economic Factors," Population Reference Bureau, January 21, 2021, https://www.prb.org/resources/high-premature-birth-rates-among-u-s-black-women-may-reflect-the-stress-of-racism-and-health-and-economic-factors/.

21 Thu T. Nguyen et al. "The Association Between State-Level Racial Attitudes Assessed From Twitter Data and Adverse Birth Outcomes: Observational Study," *JMIR Public Health Surveillance* 6, no. 3 (July 2020): e17103, https://doi.org/10.2196/17103.

22 "Quick Facts: Colorado," July 1, 2021, United States Census Bureau, https://www.census.gov/quickfacts/CO#qf-headnote-a.

23 Colorado Department of Public Health and Environment, "Recommendations to Reduce Preterm Birth in Colorado," accessed June 10, 2022, https://cdphe.colorado.gov/sites/cdphe/files/PF_Preterm-BirthRecs.pdf.

24 Jeannette R. Ickovics et al., "Group Prenatal Care and Perinatal Outcomes: A Randomized Controlled Trial," *Obstetrics & Gynecology* 110, no. 2.1 (August 2007): 330–339. https://doi.org/10.1097/01.AOG.0000275284.24298.23.

25 Elizabeth Wastnedge et al., "Interventions to Reduce Preterm Birth and Stillbirth, and Improve Outcomes for Babies Born Preterm in Low- and Middle-Income Countries: A Systematic Review," *Journal of Global Health*, no. 1 (2021), https://jogh.org/2021/jogh-11-04050.

26 Ai-Ru Chia et al., "Maternal Dietary Patterns and Birth Outcomes: A Systematic Review and Meta-Analysis," *Advances in Nutrition* 10, no. 4 (July 2019): 685–695. http://doi.org/10.1093/advances/nmy123.

27 Janette Khoury et al., "Effect of a Cholesterol-Lowering Diet on Maternal, Cord, and Neonatal Lipids, and Pregnancy Outcome: A Randomized Clinical Trial," *American Journal of Obstetrics and Gynecology* 193, no. 4 (October 2005): 1292–1301. http://doi.org/10.1016/j.ajog.2005.05.016.

28 Jane Sandall et al., "Midwife-Led Continuity Models Versus Other Models of Care for Childbearing Women," *Cochrane Database of Systematic Reviews*, no. 4 (April 2016), https://doi.org/10.1002/14651858.CD004667.pub5.

Chapter 6

1 Oneeka Williams, *Not Today Negativity!* (Newtonville, MA: Dr. Dee Dee Dynamo Books 2021), 117.

2 Oneeka Williams, Personal Communication, April 29, 2022.

3 Williams, *Not Today Negativity!*, 110.

4 Williams, *Not Today Negativity!*, 118.

5 "Multifetal Gestations Twin Triplet and Higher-Order Multifetal Pregnancies," *ACOG Practice Bulletin*, no. 231 (June 2021), https://www.acog.org/clinical/clinical-guidance/practice-bulletin/articles/2021/06/multifetal-gestations-twin-triplet-and-higher-order-multifetal-pregnancies.

6 "Twin Birth Rates in the United States between 1980 and 2019, by Ethnicity," statista, February 2022, https://www.statista.com/statistics/244913/twin-birth-rates-in-the-united-states-by-ethnicity/.

7 Gilles Pison, "Nearly Half of the World's Twins are Born in Africa," *Population et sociétés*, no. 360 (September 2000): 1–4. https://www.ined.fr/fichier/s_rubrique/18789/publi_pdf2_pop_and_soc_english_360.en.pdf.

8 Joyce A. Martin and Melissa M. Park, "Trends in Twin and Triplet Births: 1980–97," *National Vital Statistics Reports* 47, no. 24 (1999). https://www.cdc.gov/nchs/data/nvsr/nvsr47/nvs47_24.pdf.

9 Michelle J.K. Osterman et al., "Births: Final Data for 2020," *National Vital Statistics Reports* 70, no. 17 (2020), https://www.cdc.gov/nchs/data/nvsr/nvsr70/nvsr70-17.pdf.

10 Jacqueline H. Grant, Catherine J. Vladutiu, and Tracy A. Manuck, "Racial Disparities in Delivery Gestational Age among Twin Pregnancies," *American Journal of Perinatology* 34, no. 11 (2017): 1065–1071. http://doi.org/10.1055/s-0037-1603764.

11 Jose A. Rauh-Hain et al., "Risk for Developing Gestational Diabetes in Women with Twin Pregnancies," *Journal of Maternal Fetal-Neonatal Medicine* 22, no. 4 (2009): 293–299. http://doi.org/10.1080/14767050802663194.

12 William H. Goodnight and Roger B. Newman, "Optimal Nutrition for Improved Twin Pregnancy Outcome," *Obstetrics & Gynecology* 114, no. 5 (2009): 1121–1134. https://doi.org/10.1097/AOG.0b013e3181bb14c8.

13 Barbara Luke et al., "Specialized Prenatal Care and Maternal and Infant Outcomes in Twin Pregnancy," *American Journal Obstetrics and Gynecology* 189, no. 4 (October 2003): 934–938. https://doi.org/10.1067/s0002-9378(03)01054-8.

14 Luke et al., "Specialized Prenatal Care," 934–935.

15 Williams, *Not Today Negativity!*, 119.

Chapter 7

1 "Gestational Hypertension and Preeclampsia," *ACOG Practice Bulletin*, no. 222 (June 2020), https://www.acog.org/clinical/clinical-guidance/practice-bulletin/articles/2020/06/gestational-hypertension-and-preeclampsia.

2 "Chronic Hypertension in Pregnancy," *ACOG Practice Bulletin*, no. 203 (January 2019), https://www.acog.org/clinical/clinical-guidance/practice-bulletin/articles/2019/01/chronic-hypertension-in-pregnancy.

3 Lale Say et al., "Global Causes of Maternal Death: A WHO Systematic Analysis," *Lancet* 2, no. 6 (June 2014): E323, https://doi.org/10.1016/S2214-109X(14)70227-X.

4 Marian F. MacDorman et al., "Racial and Ethnic Disparities in Maternal Mortality in the United States Using Enhanced Vital Records, 2016–2017," *American Journal of Public Health* 111, no. 9 (2021): 1673–1681. https://doi.org/10.2105/AJPH.2021.306375.

5 *Report from Maternal Mortality Review Committees: A View into Their Critical Role*, 2017, https://reviewtoaction.org/national-resource/report-mmrcs-view-their-critical-role.

6 *Report from Maternal Mortality Review Committees*, 24.

7 *Report from Maternal Mortality Review Committees*, 28.

8 Katy B. Kozhimannil et al., "Association between Loss of Hospital-Based Obstetric Services and Birth Outcomes in Rural Counties in the United States," *JAMA* 319, no. 12 (2018): 1239–1247. https://doi.org/10.1001/jama.2018.1830.

9 "Why Ob-Gyns are Burning Out," American College of Obstetricians and Gynecologists, October 28, 2019, https://www.acog.org/news/news-articles/2019/10/why-ob-gyns-are-burning-out.

10 Amanda D'Ambrosio, "Black Doctor Dies After Giving Birth, Underscoring Maternal Mortality Crisis," MedPage Today, November 2, 2020, https://www.medpagetoday.com/obgyn/pregnancy/89462.

11 Achim Troja et al., "Management of Spontaneous Hepatic Rupture on Top of HELLP Syndrome: Case Report and Review of the Literature," *Viszeralmedizin* 31, no. 3 (2015): 205–208. https://doi.org/10.1159/000376601.

12 Gaurav Ghosh et al., "Racial/Ethnic Differences in Pregnancy-Related Hypertensive Disease in Nulliparous Women," *Ethnicity and Disease* 24, no. 3 (2014): 283–289. https://www.ncbi.nlm.nih.gov/pmc/articles/PMC4171100/.

13 Ellen Boakye et al., "Nativity-Related Disparities in Preeclampsia and Cardiovascular Disease Risk Among a Racially Diverse Cohort of US Women," *JAMA Network Open* 4, no. 12 (2021): e2139564. https://doi.org/10.1001/jamanetworkopen.2021.39564.

14 "U.S.-born Black Women at Higher Risk of Preeclampsia than Black Immigrants," American Heart Association Newsroom, November 9, 2020, https://newsroom.heart.org/news/u-s-born-black-women-at-higher-risk-of-preeclampsia-than-black-immigrants.

15 Elizabeth Cooney, "Predicting Preeclampsia from a Blood Test Holds Promise for Pregnancy Complications," Stat, January 5, 2022, https://www.statnews.com/2022/01/05/predicting-preeclampsia-blood-test-pregnancy-complications/; Morten Rasmussen et al., "RNA Profiles Reveal Signatures of Future Health and Disease in Pregnancy," *Nature*, no. 601 (2022): 422–427. https://doi.org/10.1038/s41586-021-04249-w.

16 "An Ounce of Prevention Is Worth a Pound of Cure," VoA Learning English, March 14, 2020, https://learningenglish.voanews.com/a/an-ounce-of-prevention-is-worth-a-pound-of-cure-/5326585.html.

17 US Preventive Services Task Force, "Aspirin Use to Prevent Preeclampsia and Related Morbidity and Mortality: US Preventive Services Task Force Recommendation Statement," *JAMA* 326, no. 12 (2021): 1186–1191. https://doi.org/10.1001/jama.2021.14781.

18 "Electronic Medical Records/Electronic Health Records (EMRs/EHRs)," Centers for Disease Control and Prevention, last updated October 14, 2021, https://www.cdc.gov/nchs/fastats/electronic-medical-records.htm.

19 Kat Jercich, "U.S. Clinicians Spend 50% More Time in EHR than Those in Other Countries," HealthcareITNews, December 17, 2020, https://www.healthcareitnews.com/news/us-clinicians-spend-50-more-time-ehr-those-other-countries.

20 Anne Lise Brantsæter et al., "A Dietary Pattern Characterized by High Intake of Vegetables, Fruits, and Vegetable Oils Is Associated with Reduced Risk of

Preeclampsia in Nulliparous Pregnant Norwegian Women," *Journal of Nutrition* 139, no. 6 (2009): 1162–1168. https://doi.org/10.3945/jn.109.104968.

21 Rebecca Allen et al., "Effect of Diet- and Lifestyle-Based Metabolic Risk-Modifying Interventions on Preeclampsia: A Meta-analysis," *Acta Obstetricia et Gynecologica Scandinavica* 93, no. 10 (October 2014): 973–985. https://doi.org/10.1111/aogs.12467.

22 Anum S. Minhas et al., "Mediterranean-Style Diet and Risk of Preeclampsia by Race in the Boston Birth Cohort," *Journal of the American Heart Association* 11, no. 9 (2022): e022589. https://doi.org/10.1161/JAHA.121.022589.

23 John La Puma, "What Is Culinary Medicine and What Does It Do?," *Population Health Management* 19, no. 1 (February 2016): 1–3. https://doi.org/10.1089/pop.2015.0003.

Chapter 8

1 "What is Stillbirth?," Center for Disease Control and Prevention, last modified November 16, 2020, https://www.cdc.gov/ncbddd/stillbirth/facts.html.

2 Shannon M. Pruitt et al., "Racial and Ethnic Disparities in Fetal Deaths—United States, 2015–2017," *Morbidity and Mortality Weekly Report Weekly* 69, no. 37 (September 18, 2020): 1277–1282. https://www.cdc.gov/mmwr/volumes/69/wr/mm6937a1.htm.

3 Elizabeth C.W. Gregory, Claudia P. Valenzuela, and Donna L. Hoyert, "Fetal Mortality: United States, 2019," *National Vital Statistics Reports* 70, no. 11 (October 26, 2021), https://www.cdc.gov/nchs/data/nvsr/nvsr70/nvsr70-11.pdf.

4 Pruitt et al., "Racial and Ethnic Disparities."

5 Gregory, Valenzuela, and Hoyert, "Fetal Mortality: United States, 2019."

6 Marian Willinger, Chia-Wen Ko, and Uma M. Reddy, "Racial Disparities in Stillbirth Risk Across Gestation in the United States," *American Journal of Obstetrics and Gynecology* 201, no. 5 (November 2009): 469.e1. https://doi.org/10.1016%2Fj.ajog.2009.06.057.

7 R. Din-Dzietham and I. Hertz-Picciotto, "Infant Mortality Difference between Whites and African Americans: The Effect of Maternal Education," *American Journal of Public Health* 88, no. 4 (1998): 651–656. https://doi.org/10.2105/AJPH.88.4.651.

8 Cheryl L. Giscombé and Marci Lobel, "Explaining Disproportionately High Rates of Adverse Birth Outcomes Among African Americans: The Impact of Stress, Racism, and Related Factors in Pregnancy," *Psychology Bulletin* 131, no. 5 (2005): 662–683. https://doi.org/10.1037/0033-2909.131.5.662.

9 Carol J.R. Hogue et al., "A Population-Based Case-Control Study of Stillbirth: The Relationship of Significant Life Events to the Racial Disparity for African Americans," *American Journal of Epidemiology* 177, no. 8 (2013): 755–767. https://doi.org/10.1093/aje/kws381.

10 William A. Grobman et al., "Labor Induction Versus Expectant Management in Low-Risk Nulliparous Women," *New England Journal of Medicine* 379 (2018): 513–523. https://doi.org/10.1056/NEJMoa1800566.

11 Zohra S. Lassi et al., "Effects of Nutritional Interventions During Pregnancy on Birth, Child Health and Development Outcomes: A Systematic Review of Evidence from Low- and Middle-Income Countries," *Campbell Systematic Reviews* 17, no. 2 (2021): e1150. https://doi.org/10.1002/cl2.1150.

12 Amanda D'Ambrosio, "High-Quality Diet Cut Risk of Fetal Growth Restriction," MedPage Today, February 3, 2022, https://www.medpagetoday.com/meetingcoverage/smfm/97015.

13 American College of Obstetricians and Gynecologists and the Society for Maternal-Fetal Medicine, "Management of Stillbirth," Obstetric Care Consensus, March 2020, https://www.acog.org/clinical/clinical-guidance/obstetric-care-consensus/articles/2020/03/management-of-stillbirth.

14 Oregon Health & Science University. "How High-Fat Diet During Pregnancy Increases Risk of Stillbirth," ScienceDaily, June 3, 2011, https://www.sciencedaily.com/releases/2011/06/110602153036.htm; Antonio E. Frias et al., "Maternal High-Fat Diet Disturbs Uteroplacental Hemodynamics and Increases the Frequency of Stillbirth in a Nonhuman Primate Model of Excess Nutrition," *Endocrinology* 152, no. 6 (June 1, 2011): 2456–2464. https://doi.org/10.1210/en.2010-1332.

15 Ruofan Yao et al., "Obesity and the Risk of Stillbirth: A Population-Based Cohort Study," *American Journal of Obstetrics and Gynecology* 210, no. 5 (May 2014): 457.e1. https://doi.org/10.1016/j.ajog.2014.01.044.

16 Erika Ota et al., "Antenatal Interventions for Preventing Stillbirth, Fetal Loss and Perinatal Death: An Overview of Cochrane Systematic Reviews," *Cochrane Database of Systematic Reviews*, no. 12 (2020), https://doi.org/10.1002/14651858.CD009599.pub2.

17 Jane Sandall et al., "Midwife-Led Continuity Models Versus Other Models of Care for Childbearing Women," *Cochrane Database of Systematic Reviews*, no. 4 (April 2016), https://doi.org/10.1002/14651858.CD004667.pub5.

18 Zohra S. Lassi and Zulfiqar A. Bhutta, "Community-Based Intervention Packages for Reducing Maternal and Neonatal Morbidity and Mortality and Improving Neonatal Outcomes," *Cochrane Database of Systematic Reviews*, no. 4 (2016), https://doi.org/10.1002/14651858.CD007754.pub3.

19 Zulfiqar A. Bhutta et al., "Improvement of Perinatal and Newborn Care in Rural Pakistan Through Community-Based Strategies: A Cluster-Randomized Effectiveness Trial," *Lancet* 377, no. 9763 (January 2011): 403–412. https://doi.org/10.1016/S0140-6736(10)62274-X.

20 Wanda Irving, Personal Communication, March 31, 2022.

21 Wanda Irving, Personal Communication, March 31, 2022.

Chapter 9

1 Mary Ann DePietro and Clarissa Stephens, "What Is the Average Baby Weight by Month?," *Medical News Today*, September 6, 2021, https://www.medicalnewstoday.com/articles/325630; "Born to Lose: How Birth Weight Affects Adult Health and Success," University of Michigan News, June 5,

2007, https://news.umich.edu/born-to-lose-how-birth-weight-affects-adult -health-and-success/.

2 Rucker C. Johnson and Robert F. Schoeni, "The Influence of Early-Life Events on Human Capital, Health Status, and Labor Market Outcomes Over the Life Course," National Poverty Center Working Paper Series, Paper No. 07-05, February 2007, http://npc.umich.edu/publications/u/working_paper05-07. pdf.

3 Lazaros Belbasis et al., "Birth Weight in Relation to Health and Disease in Later Life: An Umbrella Review of Systematic Reviews and Meta-analyses," *BMC Medicine*, no. 14 (2016): art. 147, https://doi.org/10.1186/s12916-016-0692-5.

4 Richard J. David and James W. Collins, "Differing Birth Weight among Infants of U.S.-Born Blacks, African-Born Blacks, and U.S.-Born Whites," *New England Journal of Medicine* 337, no. 17 (1997): 1209–1214. https://doi. org/10.1056/NEJM199710233371706.

5 Eugenia K. Pallotto, James W. Collins, Jr., and Richard J. David, "Enigma of Maternal Race and Infant Birth Weight: A Population-Based Study of US-Born Black and Caribbean-Born Black Women," *American Journal of Epidemiology* 151, no. 11 (June 2000): 1080–1085. https://doi.org/10.1093/oxfordjournals.aje. a010151.

6 Tanya M. Simms et al., "The Genetic Structure of Populations from Haiti and Jamaica Reflect Divergent Demographic Histories," *American Journal of Physical Anthropology* 142, no. 1 (2010): 49–66. https://doi.org/10.1002/ajpa.21194.

7 Linda Villarosa, "Why America's Black Mothers and Babies Are in a Life-or-Death Crisis," *New York Times*, April 11, 2018, https://www.nytimes. com/2018/04/11/magazine/black-mothers-babies-death-maternal-mortality. html.

8 Linda Villarosa, *Under the Skin: The Hidden Toll of Racism on American Lives and the Health of Our Nation* (New York: Doubleday, 2022).

9 "Low Birthweight," March of Dimes, last updated June 2021, https://www. marchofdimes.org/complications/low-birthweight.aspx.

10 James W. Collins, Jr., Shou-Yien Wu, and Richard J. David, "Differing Inter-generational Birth Weights among the Descendants of US-Born and For-eign-Born Whites and African Americans in Illinois," *American Journal of Epidemiology* 155, no. 3 (February 2002): 210–216. https://doi.org/10.1093/ aje/155.3.210.

11 Theresa Andrasfay and Noreen Goldman, "Intergenerational Change in Birthweight," *Epidemiology* 31, no. 5 (September 2020): 649–658. https://doi. org/10.1097/EDE.0000000000001217.

12 Tyan Parker Dominguez et al., "Differences in the Self-Reported Racism Experiences of US-Born and Foreign-Born Black Pregnant Women," *Social Science & Medicine* 69, no. 2 (2009): 258–265. https://doi.org/10.1016/j. socscimed.2009.03.022.

13 E.K. Seaton et al., "The Prevalence of Perceived Discrimination among African American and Caribbean Black Youth," *Developmental Psychology* 44, no. 5 (2008): 1288–1297. https://doi.org/10.1037/a0012747.

14 Parker Dominguez et al., "Differences in the Self-Reported Racism Experiences."

15 Jill Jin, "Babies with Low Birth Weight," *JAMA* 313, no. 4 (2015): 432. https://doi.org/10.1001/jama.2014.3698.

16 "America's Children: Key National Indicators of Well-Being, 2021: Preterm Birth and Low Birthweight," ChildStats.org, accessed May 23, 2022, https://www.childstats.gov/americaschildren/health1.asp.

17 Michelle J.K. Osterman et al., "Births: Final Data for 2020," *National Vital Statistics Reports* 70, no. 17 (February 2022), https://www.cdc.gov/nchs/data/nvsr/nvsr70/nvsr70-17.pdf.

18 Elizabeth A. Pollock et al., "Trends in Infants Born at Low Birthweight and Disparities by Maternal Race and Education from 2003 to 2018 in the United States," *BMC Public Health*, no. 21 (2021): art. 1117. https://doi.org/10.1186/s12889-021-11185-x.

19 Miriam Zoila Pérez, "How Racism Harms Pregnant Women—and What Can Help," Filmed 2016. TED video. https://www.ted.com/talks/miriam_zoila_perez_how_racism_harms_pregnant_women_and_what_can_help/transcript.

20 *The JJ WAY®: Community-Based Maternity Center Final Evaluation Report*, Visionary Vanguard Group, 2017, https://secureservercdn.net/198.71.233.72/qj7.106.myftpupload.com/wp-content/uploads/2022/03/The-JJ-Way®-Community-based-Maternity-Center-Evaluation-Report-2017-1.pdf.

21 *The JJ WAY®: Community-Based Maternity Center Final Evaluation Report*, 3.

22 Eunju Lee et al., "Reducing Low Birth Weight Through Home Visitation: A Randomized Controlled Trial," *American Journal of Preventive Medicine* 36, no. 2 (2009): 154–160. https://doi.org/10.1016/j.amepre.2008.09.029.

23 Lee et al., "Reducing Low Birth Weight Through Home Visitation," 155.

24 Lee et al., "Reducing Low Birth Weight Through Home Visitation," 156.

25 Jane S. Norbeck, Jeanne F. DeJoseph, Renée T. Smith, "A Randomized Trial of an Empirically Derived Social Support Intervention to Prevent Low Birthweight among African American Women," *Social Science & Medicine* 43, no. 6 (1996): 947–954. https://doi.org/10.1016/0277-9536(96)00003-2.

26 Norbeck, DeJoseph, and Smith, "A Randomized Trial," 948.

27 Norbeck, DeJoseph, and Smith, "A Randomized Trial," 950.

28 David L. Olds, JoAnn Robinson, Lisa Pettitt, Dennis W. Luckey, John Holmberg, Rosanna K. Ng, Kathy Isacks, Karen Sheff, and Charles R. Henderson, Jr., "Effects of Home Visits by Paraprofessionals and by Nurses: Age 4 Follow-up Results of a Randomized Trial," *Pediatrics* 114, no. 6 (2004): 1560–1568. https://doi.org/10.1542/peds.2004-0961.

29 "Female Physicians Face Higher Rates of Infertility and Pregnancy Complications," ASH Clinical News, November 2021, https://ashpublications.org/ashclinicalnews/news/1426/Female-Physicians-Face-Higher-Rates-of-Infertility.

Chapter 10

1 Heather Andrea Williams, "How Slavery Affected African American Families," Freedom's Story, TeacherServe. National Humanities Center, accessed April 24,

2022, http://nationalhumanitiescenter.org/tserve/freedom/1609-1865/essays/aafamilies.htm.

2 Steven Ruggles, "The Origins of African-American Family Structure," *American Sociological Review* 59, (February 1994): 136–151. https://users.pop.umn.edu/~ruggles/Articles/Af-Am-fam.pdf.

3 Gerald F. Goodwin, "Black and White in Vietnam," *New York Times*, July 18, 2017, https://www.nytimes.com/2017/07/18/opinion/racism-vietnam-war.html.

4 Paul Hemez and Chanell Washington, "Percentage and Number of Children Living with Two Parents Has Dropped Since 1968," United States Census Bureau, April 12, 2021, https://www.census.gov/library/stories/2021/04/number-of-children-living-only-with-their-mothers-has-doubled-in-past-50-years.html.

5 Calvina Ellerbe, "Racial Differences in Marital Outcomes among Unmarried Mothers: The Influence of Perceived Marital Benefits and Expectations," Fragile Families Working Paper no. WP18-03-FF, January 2018, https://fragilefamilies.princeton.edu/sites/fragilefamilies/files/wp18-03-ff.pdf.

6 R. Kelly Raley, Megan M. Sweeney, and Danielle Wondra, "The Growing Racial and Ethnic Divide in U.S. Marriage Patterns," *Future Child* 25, no. 2 (Fall 2015): 89–109. https://doi.org/10.1353/foc.2015.0014.

7 John Gramlich, "Black Imprisonment Rate in the U.S. Has Fallen by a Third Since 2006," Pew Research Center, May 6, 2020, https://www.pewresearch.org/fact-tank/2020/05/06/share-of-black-white-hispanic-americans-in-prison-2018-vs-2006/.

8 Gretchen Livingston and Anna Brown, "Trends and Patterns in Intermarriage," Pew Research Center, May 28, 2017, https://www.pewresearch.org/social-trends/2017/05/18/1-trends-and-patterns-in-intermarriage/.

9 Raley et al., "The Growing Racial and Ethnic Divide."

10 Livingston and Brown, "Trends and Patterns in Intermarriage."

11 Elizabeth Caucutt, Nezih Guner, and Christopher Rauh, "Incarceration, Unemployment, and the Black–White Marriage Gap in the US," VOX EU, April 6, 2019, https://voxeu.org/article/incarceration-unemployment-and-black-white-marriage-gap-us.

12 Raley et al., "The Growing Racial and Ethnic Divide."

13 Ralph Richard Banks, "Why Interracial Marriage Is Good for Black Women—and the Best Hope for Restoring Marriage in the Black Community," Council on Contemporary Families, accessed April 25, 2022, https://sites.utexas.edu/contemporaryfamilies/2011/08/30/why-interracial-marriage-is-good-for-black-women/.

14 Feroz Ahmed, "Unmarried Mothers as a High-Risk Group for Adverse Pregnancy Outcomes," *Journal of Community Health* 15, no. 1 (February 1990): 35–44. https://doi.org/10.1007/BF01350184.

15 Prakesh S. Shah, Jamie Zao, and Samana Ali, "Maternal Marital Status and Birth Outcomes: A Systematic Review and Meta-analyses," *Maternal and Child Health Journal* 15, no. 7 (2011): 1097–1109. https://doi.org/10.1007/s10995-010-0654-z.

16　Gopal K. Singh, "Trends and Social Inequalities in Maternal Mortality in the United States, 1969–2018," *International Journal of Maternal and Child Health and AIDS* 10, no. 1 (2021): 29–42. https://doi.org/10.21106/ijma.444.

17　Linda Villarosa, "Why America's Black Mothers and Babies Are in a Life-or-Death Crisis," *New York Times*, April 11, 2018, https://www.nytimes.com/2018/04/11/magazine/black-mothers-babies-death-maternal-mortality.html.

18　Meghan A. Bohren et al., "Continuous Support for Women during Childbirth," *Cochrane Database of Systematic Reviews*, no. 7 (2017), https://doi.org/10.1002/14651858.CD003766.pub6.

19　Katy B. Kozhimannil et al., "Modeling the Cost-Effectiveness of Doula Care Associated with Reductions in Preterm Birth and Cesarean Delivery," *Birth* 43, no. 1 (March 2016): 20–27. https://doi.org/10.1111/birt.12218.

20　Kenneth J. Gruber, Susan H. Cupito, and Christina F. Dobson, "Impact of Doulas on Healthy Birth Outcomes," *Journal of Perinatal Education* 22, no. 1 (Winter 2013): 49. https://doi.org/10.1891/1058-1243.22.1.49.

21　Doula Medicaid Project, National Health Law Program, accessed April 25, 2022, https://healthlaw.org/doulamedicaidproject/.

22　Mark Swartz, "The Bridgeport Baby Bundle: Thinking in Systems, not Programs," Early Learning Nation, April 15, 2021, https://earlylearningnation.com/2021/04/the-bridgeport-baby-bundle-thinking-in-systems-not-programs/.

23　New Haven Early Start, Community Foundation for Greater New Haven, accessed June 13, 2022, https://www.cfgnh.org/leading-on-issues/healthy-families/new-haven-healthy-start.

24　Zohra S. Lassi, Jai K. Das, Rehana A. Salam, and Zulfiqar A. Bhutta, "Evidence from Community Level Inputs to Improve Quality of Care for Maternal and Newborn Health: Interventions and Findings," *Reproductive Health* 11 (2014): art. S2, at 15. https://doi.org/10.1186/1742-4755-11-S2-S2.

Chapter 11

1　"Sickle Cell Disease (SCD)," Centers for Disease Control and Prevention, last updated May 25, 2022, https://www.cdc.gov/ncbddd/sicklecell/index.html.

2　"Understanding Changes in Life Expectancy," Cystic Fibrosis Foundation, accessed May 9, 2022, https://www.cff.org/managing-cf/understanding-changes-life-expectancy.

3　Sophie Lanzkron, C. Patrick Carroll, and Carlton Haywood, Jr., Mortality Rates and Age at Death from Sickle Cell Disease: U.S., 1979–2005," *Public Health Reports* 128, no. 2 (March–April 2013): 110–116. https://doi.org/10.1177/003335491312800206.

4　Lanzkron, Carroll, and Haywood, Jr., "Mortality Rates and Age at Death from Sickle Cell Disease."

5　@c.l.a.u.d.i.a.f, Instagram account, accessed March 27, 2021, https://www.instagram.com/c.l.a.u.d.i.a.f/.

6Coretta M. Jenerette, and Cheryl Brewer, "Health-Related Stigma in Young Adults with Sickle Cell Disease," *Journal of the National Medical Association* 102, no. 11 (2010): 1050–1055. https://doi.org/10.1016/s0027-9684(15)30732-x.

7Noria McCarther, Emily E. Daggett, Manesha Putra, "Racial Disparities in Severe Maternal Morbidity during Delivery Admission for People with Sickle Cell Anemia," *American Journal of Obstetrics and Gynecology* 226, no. 1 (2022): S673, https://doi.org/10.1016/j.ajog.2021.11.1111.

8Candace H. Feldman et al., "Epidemiology and Sociodemographics of Systemic Lupus Erythematosus and Lupus Nephritis among U.S. Adults with Medicaid Coverage, 2000–2004," *Arthritis Rheumatism* 65, no. 3 (March 2013): 753–763. https://doi.org/10.1002/art.37795.

9Megan E.B. Clowse, "Lupus Activity in Pregnancy," *Rheumatic Disease Clinics of North America* 33, no. 2 (2007): 237–v. https://www.ncbi.nlm.nih.gov/pmc/articles/PMC2745966/; Megan E.B. Clowse, Margaret Jamison, Evan Myers, and Andra H. James, "National Study of Medical Complications in SLE Pregnancies," *Arthritis and Rheumatism* 54, no. 9 (September 2006): P127.E1–127. E6. https://doi.org/10.1016/j.ajog.2008.03.012.

10Megan E.B. Clowse and Chad Grotegut, "Racial and Ethnic Disparities in the Pregnancies of Women With Systemic Lupus Erythematosus," *Arthritis Care Research* 68, no. 10 (October 2016): 1567–1572. https://doi.org/10.1002/acr.22847.

11Sam Roberts, "Yvette Fay Francis-McBarnette, a Pioneer in Treating Sickle Cell Anemia, Dies at 89," New York Times, April 7, 2016, https://www.nytimes.com/2016/04/08/nyregion/yvette-fay-francis-mcbarnette-a-pioneer-in-treating-sickle-cell-anemia-dies-at-89.html.

12Alison Snyder, "Yvette Fay Francis-McBarnette," *Lancet* 387, no. 10031 (May 7, 2016): 1092, https://doi.org/10.1016/S0140-6736(16)30411-1.

13Roberts, "Yvette Fay Francis-McBarnette."

14Lanetta Bronté-Hall, personal page, Foundation for Sickle Cell Disease Research, accessed June 11, 2022, https://www.fscdr.org/team/lanetta-bronte-hall/.

15Lanetta Bronté-Hall, MD, President and Chief Health Office, The Foundation for Sickle Cell Disease Research, interview by the author May 18, 2022.

16Megan Elizabeth Bowles Clowse, personal page, Department of Medicine, Duke University School of Medicine, accessed May 1, 2022, https://medicine.duke.edu/profile/megan-elizabeth-bowles-clowse.

17Megan E.B. Clowse, MD, Associate Professor, Duke University School of Medicine, interview by the author, May 2, 2022.

Chapter 12

1Daphna Motro et al., "The 'Angry Black Woman' Stereotype at Work," *Harvard Business Review*, January 31, 2022, https://hbr.org/2022/01/the-angry-black-woman-stereotype-at-work.

2Jasmine A. Abrams, Ashley Hill, and Morgan Maxwell, "Underneath the Mask of the Strong Black Woman Schema: Disentangling Influences of Strength and

Self-Silencing on Depressive Symptoms among U.S. Black Women," *Sex Roles* 80 (2019): 517–526. https://doi.org/10.1007/s11199-018-0956-y.

3 Soumyadeep Mukherjee et al., "Racial/Ethnic Disparities in Antenatal Depression in the United States: A Systematic Review," *Maternal and Child Health Journal* 20, no. 9 (September 2016): 1780–1797. https://doi.org/10.1007/s10995-016-1989-x.

4 Taghreed N. Salameh et al., "Racial/Ethnic Differences in Mental Health Treatment among a National Sample of Pregnant Women with Mental Health and/or Substance Use Disorders in the United States," *Journal of Psychosomatic Research*, no. 121 (June 2019): 74–80. https://doi.org/10.1016/j.jpsychores.2019.03.015.

5 A. Yamamoto, M.C. McCormick, and H.H. Burris, "Disparities in Antidepressant Use in Pregnancy," *Journal of Perinatology* 35 (2015): 246–251. https://doi.org/10.1038/jp.2014.197.

6 Albert L. Siu and US Preventive Services Task Force (USPSTF), "Screening for Depression in Adults: US Preventive Services Task Force Recommendation Statement," *JAMA* 315, no. 4 (January 2016): 380–387. https://doi.org/10.1001/jama.2015.18392.

7 "Mental Health Care Health Professional Shortage Areas (HPSAs)," Kaiser Family Foundation, last updated September 30, 2021, https://www.kff.org/other/state-indicator/mental-health-care-health-professional-shortage-areas-hpsas/.

8 "Over One-Third of Americans Live in Areas Lacking Mental Health Professionals," USA Facts, last updated July 14, 2021, https://usafacts.org/articles/over-one-third-of-americans-live-in-areas-lacking-mental-health-professionals/.

9 Yesenia Merino, Leslie Adams, and William J. Hall, "Implicit Bias and Mental Health Professionals: Priorities and Directions for Research," *Psychiatric Services* 69, no. 6 (2018): 723–725. https://doi.org/10.1176/appi.ps.201700294.

10 Taneasha White and Jacquelyn Johnson, "Racism in Mental Health Care: Where Are We Now?," PsychCentral, April 4, 2022, https://psychcentral.com/health/racism-in-mental-health-care.

11 Michelle van Ryn and Steven S. Fu, "Paved with Good Intentions: Do Public Health and Human Service Providers Contribute to Racial/Ethnic Disparities in Health?," *American Journal of Public Health* 93, no. 2 (February 2003): 248–255. https://doi.org/10.2105/AJPH.93.2.248.

12 Solomon, Judith, "Closing the Coverage Gap Would Improve Black Maternal Health," Center on Budget and Policy Priorities, July 26, 2021, https://www.cbpp.org/research/health/closing-the-coverage-gap-would-improve-black-maternal-health.

13 Christine H. Ou and Wendy A. Hall, "Anger in the Context of Postnatal Depression: An Integrative Review," *Birth* 45, no. 4 (December 2018): 336–346. https://doi.org/10.1111/birt.12356.

14 Ou and Hall, "Anger in the Context of Postnatal Depression," 342.

15 Ou and Hall, "Anger in the Context of Postnatal Depression," 342.

Chapter 13

1   Ayodola Adigun, "Pregnant Women not More Susceptible to COVID-19, Current Data Suggests," ABC News, June 18, 2020, https://abcnews.go.com/amp/Health/pregnant-women-susceptible-covid-19-current-data-suggests/story?id=71153309.

2   Sascha Ellington et al., "Characteristics of Women of Reproductive Age with Laboratory-Confirmed SARS-CoV-2 Infection by Pregnancy Status—United States, January 22–June 7, 2020," *Morbidity and Mortality Weekly Report* 69, no. 25 (June 26, 2020): 769–775. https://www.cdc.gov/mmwr/volumes/69/wr/mm6925a1.htm; Laura D. Zambrano et al., "Update: Characteristics of Symptomatic Women of Reproductive Age with Laboratory-Confirmed SARS-CoV-2 Infection by Pregnancy Status—United States, January 22–October 3, 2020," *Morbidity and Mortality Weekly Report* 69, no. 44 (November 6, 2020): 1641–1647. https://www.cdc.gov/mmwr/volumes/69/wr/mm6944e3.htm.

3   Laurin Kasehagen et al., "COVID-19–Associated Deaths after SARS-CoV-2 Infection During Pregnancy—Mississippi, March 1, 2020–October 6, 2021," *Morbidity and Mortality Weekly Report* 70, no. 47 (November 26, 2021): 1646–1648. https://www.cdc.gov/mmwr/volumes/70/wr/mm7047e2.htm.

4   "Maternal and Infant Characteristics Among Women with Confirmed or Presumed Cases of Coronavirus Disease (COVID-19) During Pregnancy," Centers for Disease Control and Prevention, last updated May 14, 2022, https://www.cdc.gov/nchs/covid19/technical-linkage.htm.

5   Beata Mostafavi, "COVID-19 in Pregnancy: Studying Racial Disparities and Adverse Birth Outcomes," *University of Michigan Health Lab Blog*, posted February 14, 2022, https://labblog.uofmhealth.org/rounds/covid-19-pregnancy-studying-racial-disparities-and-adverse-birth-outcomes.

6   Yasmin G. Hasbini et al., "COVID-19 is Associated with Early Emergence of Preeclampsia: Results from a Large Regional Collaborative," *American Journal of Obstetrics and Gynecology* 226, no. 1 (2022), S594–S595. https://doi.org/10.1016/j.ajog.2021.11.980; Aris T. Papageorghiou et al., "Preeclampsia and COVID-19: Results from the INTERCOVID Prospective Longitudinal Study," *American Journal of Obstetrics and Gynecology* 225, no. 3 (2021): P289.E1–289.E17. https://doi.org/10.1016/j.ajog.2021.05.014.

7   Naseem S. Miller, "COVID-19 Vaccines During Pregnancy: What Research Shows," Journalist's Resource, September 29, 2021, https://journalistsresource.org/home/covid19-vaccines-pregnancy-research/.

8   Carla L. DeSisto et al., "Risk for Stillbirth Among Women with and without COVID-19 at Delivery Hospitalization—United States, March 2020–September 2021," *Morbidity and Mortality Weekly Report* 70, no. 47 (November 26, 2021): 1640–1645. https://www.cdc.gov/mmwr/volumes/70/wr/mm7047e1.htm.

9   "COVID-19 Vaccination Considerations for Obstetric–Gynecologic Care," American College of Obstetricians and Gynecologists, last updated June 3, 2022, https://www.acog.org/clinical/clinical-guidance/practice-advisory/articles/2020/12/covid-19-vaccination-considerations-for-obstetric-gynecologic-care.

10   Yawei J. Yang et al., "Association of Gestational Age at Coronavirus Disease 2019 (COVID-19) Vaccination, History of Severe Acute Respiratory Syndrome Coronavirus 2 (SARS-CoV-2) Infection, and a Vaccine Booster Dose with Maternal and Umbilical Cord Antibody Levels at Delivery," *Obstetrics & Gynecology* 139, no. 3 (March 2022): 373–380. https://doi.org/10.1097/AOG.0000000000004693; Sivan Haia Perl, Atara Uzan-Yulzari, Hodaya Klainer, Liron Asiskovich, Michal Youngster, Ehud Rinott, and Ilan Youngster, "SARS-CoV-2–Specific Antibodies in Breast Milk after COVID-19 Vaccination of Breastfeeding Women," *JAMA* 325, no. 19 (2021): 2013–2014. https://doi.org/10.1001/jama.2021.5782.

11   Natasha B. Halasa et al., "Effectiveness of Maternal Vaccination with mRNA COVID-19 Vaccine During Pregnancy Against COVID-19–Associated Hospitalization in Infants Aged <6 Months—17 States, July 2021–January 2022," *Morbidity and Mortality Weekly Report* 71, no. 7 (February 18, 2022): 264–270. https://www.cdc.gov/mmwr/volumes/71/wr/mm7107e3.htm.

12   Hilda Razzaghi et al., "COVID-19 Vaccination Coverage Among Pregnant Women During Pregnancy—Eight Integrated Health Care Organizations, United States, December 14, 2020–May 8, 2021," *Morbidity and Mortality Weekly Report* 70, no. 24 (June 18, 2021): 895–899. https://www.cdc.gov/mmwr/volumes/70/wr/mm7024e2.htm.

13   "Society for Maternal-Fetal Medicine (SMFM) Statement: SARS-CoV-2 Vaccination in Pregnancy," Society for Maternal Fetal Medicine, December 1, 2020, https://s3.amazonaws.com/cdn.smfm.org/media/2591/SMFM_Vaccine_Statement_12-1-20_(final).pdf.

14   Emily H. Adhikari and Catherine Y. Spong, "COVID-19 Vaccination in Pregnant and Lactating Women," *JAMA* 325, no. 11 (2021): 1039–1040. https://doi.org/10.1001/jama.2021.1658.

15   "Archived Cumulative Data: Percent of Pregnant People," Centers for Disease Control and Prevention, accessed April 29, 2022, https://data.cdc.gov/Vaccinations/Archived-Cumulative-Data-Percent-of-pregnant-peopl/4ht3-nbmd/data.

16   Susan E. Smith et al., "Decision Making in Vaccine Hesitant Parents and Pregnant Women—An Integrative Review," *International Journal of Nursing Studies Advances* 4 (December 2022). https://doi.org/10.1016/j.ijnsa.2022.100062.

17   Eliz Kilich, Sara Dada, and Mark R. Francis, "Factors that Influence Vaccination Decision-Making among Pregnant Women: A Systematic Review and Meta-analysis," *PLOS One*, July 9, 2020, https://doi.org/10.1371/journal.pone.0234827.

18   Kilich, Dada, and Francis, "Factors that Influence Vaccination Decision-Making," 13.

19   Sandra Crouse Quinn et al., "Breaking Down the Monolith: Understanding Flu Vaccine Uptake among African Americans," *SSM—Population Health* 4 (2018): 25–36. https://doi.org/10.1016/j.ssmph.2017.11.003.

20   Matthew Z. Dudley et al., "Racial/Ethnic Disparities in Maternal Vaccine Knowledge, Attitudes, and Intentions," *Public Health Reports* 136, no. 6 (November–December 2021): 699–709. https://doi.org/10.1177/0033354920974660.

Chapter 14

1 "Safe Prevention of the Primary Cesarean Delivery," *Obstetrics Care Consensus*, no. 1, March 2014, https://www.acog.org/clinical/clinical-guidance/obstetric-care-consensus/articles/2014/03/safe-prevention-of-the-primary-Cesarean-delivery.

2 Kevin Jacob and Jacob E. Hoerter, *Caput Succedaneum* (StatPearls Publishing, 2022). https://www.ncbi.nlm.nih.gov/books/NBK574534/.

3 "Delivery Method," March of Dimes, updated January 2022, https://www.marchofdimes.org/peristats/data?reg=99&top=8&stop=356&lev=1&slev=1&obj=1.

4 Joyce A. Martin, Brady E. Hamilton, and Michelle J.K. Osterman, "Births in the United States, *NCHS Data Brief*, no. 418 (September 2021), https://www.cdc.gov/nchs/data/databriefs/db418.pdf.

5 Laurens Holmes Jr. et al. "Implication of Vaginal and Cesarean Section Delivery Method in Black–White Differentials in Infant Mortality in the United States: Linked Birth/Infant Death Records, 2007–2016." *International Journal of Environmental Research and Public Health* 17, no. 9 (2020): 3146. https://doi.org/10.3390/ijerph17093146.

6 "Vaginal Birth After Cesarean Delivery," ACOG *Practice Bulletin*, no. 205 (February 2019), https://www.acog.org/clinical/clinical-guidance/practice-bulletin/articles/2019/02/vaginal-birth-after-Cesarean-delivery.

7 "Charles Johnson Shares the Tragic Story of His Wife Kira's Death Hours after Giving Birth," YouTube, June 7, 2018, https://youtu.be/05uBCBfrY4g.

8 "Better Data and Better Outcomes: Reducing Maternal Mortality in the U.S.," Testimony of Charles Johnson IV, Husband of the Late Kira Johnson, Founder of 4Kira4Moms, Advocate for Improved Maternal Health Policies, before the Subcommittee on Health, Committee on Energy and Commerce, U.S. House of Representatives, September 27, 2018, https://docs.house.gov/meetings/IF/IF14/20180927/108724/HHRG-115-IF14-Wstate-JohnsonC-20180927.pdf.

9 Cheri Mossburg and Taylor Romine, "Widower of Black Woman Who Died Hours after Childbirth Files Civil Rights Lawsuit against Cedars-Sinai," CNN, May 6, 2022, https://www.cnn.com/2022/05/06/us/california-civil-rights-lawsuit-cedars-sinai/index.html.

10 Elizabeth A. Howell, "Reducing Disparities in Severe Maternal Morbidity and Mortality," *Clinical Obstetrics and Gynecology* 61, no. 2 (June 2018): 387. https://doi.org/10.1097/GRF.0000000000000349.

11 Fay Menacker and Brady E. Hamilton, "Recent Trends in Cesarean Delivery in the United States," *NCHS Data Brief*, no. 35 (March 2010), https://www.cdc.gov/nchs/data/databriefs/db35.pdf.

12 "Maternal Mortality—United States, 1982–1996," *Morbidity and Mortality Weekly Report* 47, no. 34 (September 4, 1998): 705–707. https://www.cdc.gov/mmwr/preview/mmwrhtml/00054602.htm. Note that when referring to White or Black women in the book, I specifically refer to non-Hispanic White and non-Hispanic Black women.

13 Donna L. Hoyert, "Maternal Mortality Rates in the United States, 2020," National Center for Health Statistics, Centers for Disease Control and

Prevention, last updated February 23, 2022, https://www.cdc.gov/nchs/data/hestat/maternal-mortality/2020/maternal-mortality-rates-2020.htm.

14 Menacker and Hamilton, "Recent Trends in Cesarean Delivery in the United States."

15 Anna S. Leung, Eleanor K. Leung, and Richard H. Paul, "Uterine Rupture after Previous Cesarean Delivery: Maternal and Fetal Consequences," *American Journal of Obstetrics and Gynecology* 69, no. 4 (October 1993): 945–950, https://doi.org/10.1016/0002-9378(93)90032-E.

16 Benjamin P. Sachs, Cindy Kobelin, Mary Ames Castro, and Fredric Frigoletto, "The Risks of Lowering the Cesarean-Delivery Rate," *New England Journal of Medicine*, no. 340 (January 1999): 54–57. https://doi.org/10.1056/NEJM199901073400112.

17 Mona Lydon-Rochelle, Victoria L. Holt, Thomas R. Easterling, and Diane P. Martin, "Risk of Uterine Rupture during Labor among Women with a Prior Cesarean Delivery," *New England Journal of Medicine*, no. 345 (July 2001): 3–8. https://doi.org/10.1056/NEJM200107053450101.

18 "ACOG Committee on Ethics Number 289, November 2003: Surgery and Patient Choice: The Ethics of Decision Making," *Obstetrics & Gynecology* 102, no. 5 (November 2003): 1101–1106. https://doi.org/10.1016/j.obstetgynecol.2003.09.030.

19 "Caesarean Sections Should only Be Performed When Medically Necessary Says WHO," World Health Organization News, April 9, 2015, https://www.who.int/news/item/09-04-2015-caesarean-sections-should-only-be-performed-when-medically-necessary-says-who.

20 Kimberly D. Gregory, Sherri Jackson, Lisa Korst, and Moshe Fridman, "Cesarean Versus Vaginal Delivery: Whose Risks? Whose Benefits?," *American Journal Perinatology* 29, no. 1 (2012): 7–18. https://doi.org/10.1055/s-0031-1285829.

21 C.Y. Spong, M. Beall, D. Rodrigues, and M.G. Ross, "An Objective Definition of Shoulder Dystocia: Prolonged Head-to-Body Delivery Intervals and/or the Use of Ancillary Obstetric Maneuvers," *Obstetrics & Gynecology* 86, no. 3 (1995): 433–436. https://doi.org/10.1016/0029-7844(95)00188-W.

22 Oonagh E. Keag, Jane E. Norman, and Sarah J. Stock, "Long-Term Risks and Benefits Associated With Cesarean Delivery for Mother, Baby, and Subsequent Pregnancies: Systematic Review and Meta-analysis," *PLoS Medicine* 15, no. 1 (2018): e1002494. https://doi.org/10.1371/journal.pmed.1002494.

23 Rob Haskell, "Serena Williams on Motherhood, Miscarriage and Making Her Comeback," *Vogue*, January 10, 2018. https://www.vogue.com/article/serena-williams-vogue-cover-interview-february-2018.

24 Serena Williams, "How Serena Williams Saved Her Own Life," *Elle*, April 25, 2022, https://www.elle.com/life-love/a39586444/how-serena-williams-saved-her-own-life/S.

25 Emma L. Barber, Lisbet Lundsberg, and Kathleen Belanger, "Contributing Indications to the Rising Cesarean Delivery Rate," *Obstetrics & Gynecology* 118, no. 1 (July 2011): 29–38. https://doi.org/10.1097/AOG.0b013e31821e5f65.

26 "Safe Prevention of the Primary Cesarean Delivery."

27 Barber, Lundsberg, and Belanger, "Contributing Indications to the Rising Cesarean Delivery Rate."

28 Marco Huesch and Jason N. Doctor, "Factors Associated with Increased
    Cesarean Section Risk Among African American Women: Evidence from
    California, 2010," *American Journal of Public Health* 105, no. 5 (May 2015):
    956. https://doi.org/10.2105/AJPH.2014.302381.

29 Huesch and Doctor, "Factors Associated with Increased Cesarean Section
    Risk."

30 Chloë FitzGerald and Samia Hurst, "Implicit Bias in Healthcare Professionals:
    A Systematic Review," *BMC Medical Ethics*, no. 18 (2017): art. 19. https://doi.
    org/10.1186/s12910-017-0179-8.

31 Huesch and Doctor, "Factors Associated with Increased Cesarean Section
    Risk."

32 Huesch and Doctor, "Factors Associated with Increased Cesarean Section
    Risk," 960.

33 Tatyana Ali, "'Birthright': Tatyana Ali's Heartfelt Essay on the Impor-
    tance and Beauty of a Black Woman's Pregnancy Journey," *Essence*,
    November 3, 2020, https://www.essence.com/lifestyle/health-wellness/
    tatyana-ali-essay-birthright-black-maternal-health-pregnancy-motherhood/.

34 Michelle P. Debbink et al., "Racial and Ethnic Inequities in Cesarean Birth
    and Maternal Morbidity in a Low-Risk, Nulliparous Cohort," *Obstetrics
    & Gynecology* 139, no. 1 (January 2022): 73–82. https://doi.org/10.1097/
    AOG.0000000000004620.

35 Vivienne Souter et al., "Comparison of Midwifery and Obstetric Care in Low-
    Risk Hospital Births," *Obstetrics & Gynecology* 134, no. 5 (November 2019):
    1056–1065. https://doi.org/10.1097/AOG.0000000000003521.

36 Jane Sandall et al., "Midwife-Led Continuity Models Versus Other Models of
    Care for Childbearing Women," *Cochrane Database of Systematic Reviews*, no.
    4 (April 2016), https://doi.org/10.1002/14651858.CD004667.pub5.

37 "Safe Prevention of the Primary Cesarean Delivery."

38 David B. Nelson and Catherine Y. Spong, "Initiatives to Reduce Cesarean
    Delivery Rates for Low-Risk First Births," *JAMA* 325, no. 16 (2021): 1616–1617.
    https:/doi.org/10.1001/jama.2021.0084.

39 Melissa G. Rosenstein et al., "Hospital Quality Improvement Interventions,
    Statewide Policy Initiatives, and Rates of Cesarean Delivery for Nulliparous,
    Term, Singleton, Vertex Births in California," *JAMA* 325, no. 16 (2021): 1631–
    1639. https:/doi.org/10.1001/jama.2021.3816.

40 "Birth Equity," California Maternity Quality Care Collaboration, accessed
    March 16, 2022, https://www.cmqcc.org/content/birth-equity.

Chapter 15

1 Steven Carlson and Zoë Neuberger, "WIC Works: Addressing the Nutrition
   and Health Needs of Low-Income Families for More Than Four Decades,"
   Center on Budget and Policy Priorities, January 27, 2021, https://www.cbpp.
   org/research/food-assistance/wic-works-addressing-the-nutrition-and-
   health-needs-of-low-income-families.

2   Nina Martin and Renee Montagne, "Black Mothers Keep Dying After Giving Birth. Shalon Irving's Story Explains Why," NPR, December 7, 2017, https://www.npr.org/2017/12/07/568948782/black-mothers-keep-dying-after-giving-birth-shalon-irvings-story-explains-why.

3   Martin and Montagne, "Black Mothers Keep Dying After Giving Birth."

4   Roosa Tikkanen et al., "Maternal Mortality and Maternity Care in the United States Compared to 10 Other Developed Countries," Commonwealth Fund, November 18, 2020, https://www.commonwealthfund.org/publications/issue-briefs/2020/nov/maternal-mortality-maternity-care-us-compared-10-countries; Emily E. Petersen et al., "Vital Signs: Pregnancy-Related Deaths, United States, 2011–2015, and Strategies for Prevention, 13 States, 2013–2017," Morbidity and Mortality Weekly Report 68, no. 18 (May 10, 2019): 423–429. https://www.cdc.gov/mmwr/volumes/68/wr/mm6818e1.htm.

5   "Cardiomyopathy," Centers for Disease Control and Prevention, last updated December 9, 2019, https://www.cdc.gov/heartdisease/cardiomyopathy.htm.

6   Martin and Montagne, "Black Mothers Keep Dying After Giving Birth."

7   Monique Rainford, "America's Maternal Nightmare," Filmed September 27, 2018, TED video, https://www.ted.com/talks/monique_rainford_america_s_maternal_nightmare.

8   Judith Solomon, "Closing the Coverage Gap Would Improve Black Maternal Health," Center on Budget and Policy Priorities, July 26, 2021, https://www.cbpp.org/research/health/closing-the-coverage-gap-would-improve-black-maternal-health.

9   Kayla Holgash and Martha Heberlein, "Physician Acceptance of New Medicaid Patients: What Matters and What Doesn't," Health Affairs, April 10, 2019, https://doi.org/10.1377/forefront.20190401.678690; Chima D. Ndumele, Michael S. Cohen, and Paul D. Cleary, "Association of State Access Standards with Accessibility to Specialists for Medicaid Managed Care Enrollees," JAMA Internal Medicine 177, no. 10 (2017): 1445–1451. https://jamanetwork.com/journals/jamainternalmedicine/fullarticle/2648744.

10 "Optimizing Postpartum Care," Committee Opinion, no. 736 (May 2018), https://www.acog.org/clinical/clinical-guidance/committee-opinion/articles/2018/05/optimizing-postpartum-care.

11 Tikkanen et al., "Maternal Mortality and Maternity Care in the United States."

12 Tikkanen et al., "Maternal Mortality and Maternity Care in the United States."

13 "Extend Postpartum Medicaid Coverage," American College of Obstetricians and Gynecologists, accessed April 10, 2022, https://www.acog.org/advocacy/policy-priorities/extend-postpartum-medicaid-coverage.

14 Erica L. Eliason, "Adoption of Medicaid Expansion is Associated with Lower Maternal Mortality," Women's Health Issues 30, no. 3 (May 2020): 147–152. https://doi.org/10.1016/j.whi.2020.01.005.

Chapter 16

1   "Infant Mortality," Centers for Disease Control and Prevention, last updated June 22, 2022, https://www.cdc.gov/reproductivehealth/maternalinfanthealth/infantmortality.htm.

2   Danielle M. Ely and Anne K. Driscoll, "Infant Mortality in the United States, 2018: Data from the Period Linked Birth/Infant Death File," *National Vital Statistics Reports* 69, no. 7 (July 16, 2020), https://www.cdc.gov/nchs/data/nvsr/nvsr69/NVSR-69-7-508.pdf.

3   Ely and Driscoll, "Infant Mortality in the United States, 2018."

4   "Current Trends Infant Mortality—United States, 1992," *Morbidity and Mortality Weekly Report Weekly* 43, no. 49 (December 16, 1994): 905–909. https://www.cdc.gov/mmwr/preview/mmwrhtml/00033948.htm.

5   Brad N. Greenwood et al., "Patient Racial Concordance and Disparities in Birthing Mortality for Newborns," *Proceedings of the National Academy of Sciences* 117, no. 35 (2020): 21194–21200. https://doi.org/10.1073/pnas.1913405117.

6   "About TeamSTEPPS," Agency for Healthcare Research and Quality, last updated June 2019, https://www.ahrq.gov/teamstepps/about-teamstepps/index.html.

7   Antay L. Parker, Lydia L. Forsythe, and Ingrid K. Kohlmorgen, "TeamSTEPPS®: An Evidence-Based Approach to Reduce Clinical Errors Threatening Safety in Outpatient Settings: An Integrative Review," *Journal of Healthcare Risk Management* 38, no. 4 (April 2019): 19–31. https://doi.org/10.1002/jhrm.21352.

8   Ely and Driscoll, "Infant Mortality in the United States, 2018."

9   "Infant Mortality and African Americans," U.S. Department of Health and Human Services, Office of Minority Health, last updated July 8, 2021. https://minorityhealth.hhs.gov/omh/browse.aspx?lvl=4&lvlid=23.

10 Kawai O. Tanabe and Fern R. Hauck, "A United States Perspective," in *SIDS Sudden Infant and Early Childhood Death: The Past, the Present and the Future*, ed. Jhodie R. Duncan and Roger W. Byard (Adelaide: University of Adelaide Press, 2018), https://www.ncbi.nlm.nih.gov/books/NBK513376/.

11 Tanabe and Hauck, "A United States Perspective."

12 Linda Y. Fu, Rachel Y. Moon, and Fern R. Hauck, "Bed Sharing among Black Infants and Sudden Infant Death Syndrome: Interactions with Other Known Risk Factors," *Prevention* 10, no. 6 (November 2010): 376–382. https://doi.org/10.1016/j.acap.2010.09.001.

13 Brandi L. Joyner et al., "Where Should My Baby Sleep: A Qualitative Study of African American Infant Sleep Location Decisions," *Journal of the National Medical Association* 102, no. 10 (2010): 881–889. https://doi.org/10.1016/S0027-9684(15)30706-9.

14 "Sudden Unexpected Infant Death and Sudden Infant Death Syndrome," Centers for Disease Control and Prevention, last updated June 21, 2022, https://www.cdc.gov/sids/data.htm.

15 Joel Schumacher dir., *A Time to Kill* (Warner Brothers, 1996).

The Ray of Hope

1 H.R.1318—Preventing Maternal Deaths Act of 2018, 115th Cong. (2017–2018), https://www.congress.gov/bill/115th-congress/house-bill/1318/text.

2 "Analysis of Federal Bills to Strengthen Maternal Health Care," Women's Health Policy, Kaiser Family Foundation, December 21, 2020, https://www.kff.org/womens-health-policy/fact-sheet/analysis-of-federal-bills-to-strengthen-maternal-health-care/.

3 H.R.4387—Maternal Health Quality Improvement Act of 2021, 117th Cong. (2021–2022), https://www.congress.gov/bill/117th-congress/house-bill/4387; "ACOG Celebrates Long Overdue Passage of the Maternal Health Quality Improvement Act," News Release, American College of Obstetricians and Gynecologists, March 11, 2022, https://www.acog.org/news/news-releases/2022/03/acog-celebrates-passage-of-maternal-health-quality-improvement-act.

4 H.R.959–Black Maternal Health Momnibus Act of 2021, 117th Cong. (2021–2022), https://www.congress.gov/bill/117th-congress/house-bill/959.

5 "Momnibus," Black Maternal Health Caucus, accessed June 8, 2022, https://blackmaternalhealthcaucus-underwood.house.gov/Momnibus.

6 "Fact Sheet: Biden–Harris Administration Announces Additional Actions in Response to Vice President Harris's Call to Action on Maternal Health," White House, April 13, 2022, https://www.whitehouse.gov/briefing-room/statements-releases/2022/04/13/fact-sheet-biden-harris-administration-announces-additional-actions-in-response-to-vice-president-harriss-call-to-action-on-maternal-health/.

7 "Fact Sheet: Vice President Kamala Harris Announces Call to Action to Reduce Maternal Mortality and Morbidity," White House, December 7, 2021, https://www.whitehouse.gov/briefing-room/statements-releases/2021/12/07/fact-sheet-vice-president-kamala-harris-announces-call-to-action-to-reduce-maternal-mortality-and-morbidity/.

8 Usha Ranji, Ivette Gomez, and Alina Salganicoff, "Expanding Postpartum Medicaid Coverage," Women's Health Policy, Kaiser Family Foundation, March 9, 2021, https://www.kff.org/womens-health-policy/issue-brief/expanding-postpartum-medicaid-coverage/.

9 Dr. Shalon's Maternal Action Project, accessed June 4, 2022, https://www.drshalonsmap.org/.

10 Believe Her: Black Maternal Peer Support, accessed June 4, 2022, https://believeherapp.com.

11 "Haywood Brown, MD Becomes 68th President of ACOG," Duke Obstetrics & Gynecology, May 9, 2017, https://obgyn.duke.edu/news/haywood-brown-md-becomes-68th-president-acog.

12 "What We Do," National Birth Equity Collaborative, accessed June 5, 2022, https://birthequity.org/what-we-do/.

13 *The Resident*, Season 2 episode 20, "If Not Now When," directed by Rob Corn, featuring Malcome Jamal-Warner, Manish Dayal, and Shaunette Renee Wilson, aired April 15, 2019, on Fox.

14 https://blackmamasmatter.org, accessed June 5, 2022

15 Black Maternal Health Week, accessed June 5, 2022, https://blackmamasmat ter.org/bmhw/.

16 "Our Story," Nurturely, accessed June 5, 2022, https://nurturely.org/mission/.

17 Sabia C. Wade, accessed June 5, 2022, https://www.sabiawade.com.

18 Neel Shah, MD, MPP, Assistant Professor, Harvard Medical School, June 6, 2022, https://scholar.harvard.edu/shah/home.

19 Earth's Natural Touch, accessed June 6, 2022, https://earthsnaturaltouch. com/.

20 "Health Literacy Universal Precautions Toolkit, 2nd Edition," Agency for Healthcare Research and Quality, last updated September 2020, https://www. ahrq.gov/health-literacy/improve/precautions/tool2b.html.

21 Molly C. Kalmoe et al., "Physician Suicide: A Call to Action," *Missouri Medicine* 116, no. 3 (2019): 211–216. https://www.ncbi.nlm.nih.gov/pmc/articles/ PMC6690303/; Eva S. Schernhammer and Graham A. Colditz, "Suicide Rates among Physicians: A Quantitative and Gender Assessment (Meta-analysis)," *American Journal of Psychiatry* 161, no. 12 (December 2004): 2295–2302. https://doi.org/10.1176/appi.ajp.161.12.2295.

22 Leslie Kane, "'Death by 1000 Cuts': Medscape National Physician Burnout & Suicide Report 2021," Medscape, January 22, 2021, https://www.medscape. com/slideshow/2021-lifestyle-burnout-6013456.

23 Karen A. Scott, MD, MPH, FACOG, Founding CEO and Owner, Birthing Cultural Rigor, LLC, Public Health Institute, accessed June 5, 2022, https://www. phi.org/experts/karen-a-scott/.

24 SACRED Birth during COVID19, University of California San Francisco, accessed June 6, 2022, https://sacredbirth.ucsf.edu/.

25 Emily White VanGompel et al., "Psychometric Validation of a Patient-Reported Experience Measure of Obstetric Racism© (The PREM-OB Scale™ Suite)," *Birth* (March 17, 2022): 514–525. https://doi.org/10.1111/birt.12622.

26 White VanGompel et al., "Psychometric Validation of a Patient-Reported Experience."

27 Monique Rainford, "America's Maternal Nightmare," Filmed September 27, 2018, TED video, https://www.ted.com/talks/monique_rainford_america_s_ maternal_nightmare.

Bibliography

@c.l.a.u.d.i.a.f, Instagram account, accessed March 27, 2021, https://www.instagram.com/c.l.a.u.d.i.a.f/.

#lifestylemed2018, Twitter, last accessed April 17, 2022. https://twitter.com/hashtag/lifestylemed2018?src=hash.

"2021 March of Dimes Report Card," March of Dimes, 2021, https://www.marchofdimes.org/materials/March-of-Dimes-2021-Full-Report-Card.pdf.

"About Me," Ashlee Wisdom, accessed June 4, 2022, https://www.ashleewisdom.com/about-me.

"About TeamSTEPPS," Agency for Healthcare Research and Quality, last updated June 2019, https://www.ahrq.gov/teamstepps/about-teamstepps/index.html.

Abrams, Jasmine A., Ashley Hill, and Morgan Maxwell, "Underneath the Mask of the Strong Black Woman Schema: Disentangling Influences of Strength and Self-Silencing on Depressive Symptoms among U.S. Black Women," *Sex Roles* 80 (2019): 517–526. https://doi.org/10.1007/s11199-018-0956-y.

"ACOG Celebrates Long Overdue Passage of the Maternal Health Quality Improvement Act," News Release, American College of Obstetricians and Gynecologists, March 11, 2022, https://www.acog.org/news/news-releases/2022/03/acog-celebrates-passage-of-maternal-health-quality-improvement-act.

"ACOG Committee on Ethics Number 289, November 2003: Surgery and Patient Choice: The Ethics of Decision Making," *Obstetrics & Gynecology* 102, no. 5 (November 2003): 1101–1106. https://doi.org/10.1016/j.obstetgynecol.2003.09.030.

Adhikari, Emily H. and Catherine Y. Spong, "COVID-19 Vaccination in Pregnant and Lactating Women," *JAMA* 325, no. 11 (2021): 1039–1040. https://doi.org/10.1001/jama.2021.1658.

Adigun, Ayodola, "Pregnant Women not More Susceptible to COVID-19, Current Data Suggests," ABC News, June 18, 2020, https://abcnews.go.com/amp/Health/pregnant-women-susceptible-covid-19-current-data-suggests/story?id=71153309.

Ahmed, Feroz, "Unmarried Mothers as a High-Risk Group for Adverse Pregnancy Outcomes," *Journal of Community Health* 15, no. 1 (February 1990): 35–44. https://doi.org/10.1007/BF01350184.

Ali, Tatyana, "'Birthright': Tatyana Ali's Heartfelt Essay on the Importance and Beauty of a Black Woman's Pregnancy Journey," *Essence*, November 3, 2020, https://www.essence.com/lifestyle/health-wellness/tatyana-ali-essay-birthright-black-maternal-health-pregnancy-motherhood/.

Allen, Rebecca, Ewelina Rogozinska, Priya Sivarajasingam, Khalid S. Khan, and Shakila Thangaratinam, "Effect of Diet- and Lifestyle-Based Metabolic Risk-Modifying Interventions on Preeclampsia: A Meta-analysis," *Acta Obstetricia et Gynecologica Scandinavica* 93, no. 10 (October 2014): 973–985. https://doi.org/10.1111/aogs.12467.

"America's Children: Key National Indicators of Well-Being, 2021: Preterm Birth and Low Birthweight," ChildStats.org, accessed May 23, 2022, https://www.childstats.gov/americaschildren/health1.asp.

"An Ounce of Prevention Is Worth a Pound of Cure," VoA Learning English, March 14, 2020, https://learningenglish.voanews.com/a/an-ounce-of-prevention-is-worth-a-pound-of-cure-/5326585.html.

"Analysis of Federal Bills to Strengthen Maternal Health Care," Women's Health Policy, Kaiser Family Foundation, December 21, 2020, https://www.kff.org/womens-health-policy/fact-sheet/analysis-of-federal-bills-to-strengthen-maternal-health-care/.

Andrasfay, Theresa, and Noreen Goldman, "Intergenerational Change in Birthweight," *Epidemiology* 31, no. 5 (September 2020): 649–658. https://doi.org/10.1097/EDE.0000000000001217.

"Archived Cumulative Data: Percent of Pregnant People," Centers for Disease Control and Prevention, accessed April 29, 2022, https://data.cdc.gov/Vaccinations/Archived-Cumulative-Data-Percent-of-pregnant-peopl/4ht3-nbmd/data.

Bailey, Zinzi D., Nancy Krieger, Madina Agénor, Jasmine Graves, Natalia Linos, and Mary T. Bassett, "Structural Racism and Health Inequities in the USA," *Lancet* 389, no. 10077 (April 2017): 1453–1463. https://doi.org/10.1016/S0140-6736(17)30569-X.

Banks, Ralph Richard, "Why Interracial Marriage Is Good for Black Women—and the Best Hope for Restoring Marriage in the Black Community," Council on Contemporary Families, accessed April 25, 2022, https://sites.utexas.edu/contemporaryfamilies/2011/08/30/why-interracial-marriage-is-good-for-black-women/.

Barber, Emma L., Lisbet Lundsberg, and Kathleen Belanger, "Contributing Indications to the Rising Cesarean Delivery Rate," *Obstetrics & Gynecology* 118, no. 1 (July 2011): 29–38. https://doi.org/10.1097/AOG.0b013e31821e5f65.

Beata Mostafavi, "COVID-19 in Pregnancy: Studying Racial Disparities and Adverse Birth Outcomes," University of Michigan Health Lab Blog, posted February 14, 2022, https://labblog.uofmhealth.org/rounds/covid-19-pregnancy-studying-racial-disparities-and-adverse-birth-outcomes.

Belbasis, Lazaros, Makrina D. Savvidou, Chidimma Kanu, Evangelos Evangelou & Ioanna Tzoulaki, "Birth Weight in Relation to Health and Disease in Later Life: An Umbrella Review of Systematic Reviews and Meta-analyses," *BMC Medicine*, no. 14 (2016): art. 147. https://doi.org/10.1186/s12916-016-0692-5.

Believe Her: Black Maternal Peer Support, accessed June 4, 2022, https://believeherapp.com.

"Better Data and Better Outcomes: Reducing Maternal Mortality in the U.S.," Testimony of Charles Johnson IV, Husband of the Late Kira Johnson, Founder of 4Kira4Moms, Advocate for Improved Maternal Health Policies, before the Subcommittee on Health,

Committee on Energy and Commerce, U.S. House of Representatives, September 27, 2018, https://docs.house.gov/meetings/IF/IF14/20180927/108724/HHRG-115-IF14-Wstate-JohnsonC-20180927.pdf.

Bhutta, Zulfiqar A., Sajid Soofi, Simon Cousens, Shah Mohammad, Zahid A. Memon, Imran Ali, Asher Feroze, Farrukh Raza, Amanullah Khan, Steve Wall, and Jose Martines, "Improvement of Perinatal and Newborn Care in Rural Pakistan through Community-Based Strategies: A Cluster-Randomized Effectiveness Trial," *Lancet* 377, no. 9763 (January 2011): 403–412. https://doi.org/10.1016/S0140-6736(10)62274-X.

"Birth Equity," California Maternity Quality Care Collaboration, accessed March 16, 2022, https://www.cmqcc.org/content/birth-equity.

Black Maternal Health Week, accessed June 5, 2022, https://blackmamasmatter.org/bmhw/.

"Black Women & the Pay Gap," American Association of University Women, accessed June 10, 2022, https://www.aauw.org/resources/article/black-women-and-the-pay-gap/.

Blynn, Jamie, "Gabrielle Union on Infertility, Surrogacy: 'Every Route to Parenthood is Perfect,'" Today, January 23, 2019, https://www.today.com/parents/gabrielle-union-infertility-surrogacy-new-baby-girl-t147325.

Bohren, Meghan, Justus Hofmeyr, Carol Sakala, Rieko K. Fukuzawa, and Anna Cuthbert, "Continuous Support for Women during Childbirth," *Cochrane Database of Systematic Reviews*, no. 7 (2017), https://doi.org/10.1002/14651858.CD003766.pub6.

"Born to Lose: How Birth Weight Affects Adult Health and Success," University of Michigan News, June 5, 2007, https://news.umich.edu/born-to-lose-how-birth-weight-affects-adult-health-and-success/.

Borrero, Sonya B., Matthew F. Reeves, Eleanor B. Schwarz, James E. Bost, Mitchell D. Creinin, and Said A. Ibrahim, "Race, Insurance Status, and Desire for Tubal Sterilization Reversal," *Fertil Steril* 90, no. 2 (August 2008): 272–277. https://doi.org/10.1016/j.fertnstert.2007.06.041.

Brandt, Lars P. A., and Claus V. Nielsen, "Job Stress and Adverse Outcome of Pregnancy: A Causal Link or Recall Bias?," *American Journal of Epidemiology* 135, no. 3 (1992): 302–311. https://doi.org/10.1093/oxfordjournals.aje.a116284.

Brantsæter, Anne Lise, Margaretha Haugen, Sven Ove Samuelsen, Hanne Torjusen, Lill Trogstad, Jan Alexander, Per Magnus, and Helle Margrete Meltzer, "A Dietary Pattern Characterized by High Intake of Vegetables, Fruits, and Vegetable Oils Is Associated with Reduced Risk of Preeclampsia in Nulliparous Pregnant Norwegian Women," *Journal of Nutrition* 139, no. 6 (2009): 1162–1168. https://doi.org/10.3945/jn.109.104968.

Bronté-Hall, Lanetta, personal page, Foundation for Sickle Cell Disease Research, accessed June 11, 2022, https://www.fscdr.org/team/lanetta-bronte-hall/.

"Caesarean Sections Should Only Be Performed When Medically Necessary Says WHO," World Health Organization News, April 9, 2015, https://www.who.int/news/item/09-04-2015-caesarean-sections-should-only-be-performed-when-medically-necessary-says-who.

"Cardiomyopathy," Centers for Disease Control and Prevention, last updated December 9, 2019, https://www.cdc.gov/heartdisease/cardiomyopathy.htm.

Carlson, Steven, and Zoë Neuberger, "WIC Works: Addressing the Nutrition and Health Needs of Low-Income Families for More Than Four Decades," Center on Budget and Policy Priorities, January 27, 2021, https://www.cbpp.org/research/food-assistance/wic-works-addressing-the-nutrition-and-health-needs-of-low-income-families.

Caucutt, Elizabeth, Nezih Guner, and Christopher Rauh, "Incarceration, Unemployment, and the Black–White Marriage Gap in the US," VOX EU, April 6, 2019, https://voxeu.org/article/incarceration-unemployment-and-black-white-marriage-gap-us.

Chapman, Elizabeth N., Anna Kaatz, and Molly Carnes, "Physicians and Implicit Bias: How Doctors May Unwittingly Perpetuate Health Care Disparities," *Journal of General Internal Medicine* 28, no. 11 (November 2013): 1504–1510. https://doi.org/10.1007/s11606-013-2441-1.

"Charles Johnson Shares the Tragic Story of His Wife Kira's Death Hours after Giving Birth," YouTube, June 7, 2018, https://youtube/05uBCBfrY4g.

Chia, Ai-Ru, Ling-Wei Chen, Jun Shi Lai, Chun Hong Wong, Nithya Neelakantan, Rob Martinus van Dam, and Mary Foong-Fong Chong, "Maternal Dietary Patterns and Birth Outcomes: A Systematic Review and Meta-Analysis," *Advances in Nutrition* 10, no. 4 (July 2019): 685–695. http://doi.org/10.1093/advances/nmy123.

"Chronic Hypertension in Pregnancy," *Practice Bulletin*, no. 203 (January 2019), https://www.acog.org/clinical/clinical-guidance/practice-bulletin/articles/2019/01/chronic-hypertension-in-pregnancy.

Chuck, Elizabeth, "'An Amazing First Step': Advocates Hail Congress's Maternal Mortality Prevention Bill," NBC News, December 19, 2018, https://www.nbcnews.com/news/us-news/amazing-first-step-advocates-hail-congress-s-maternal-mortality-prevention-n948951.

Clowse, Megan E. B., (personal web page), Department of Medicine, Duke University School of Medicine, accessed May 1, 2022, https://medicine.duke.edu/profile/megan-elizabeth-bowles-clowse.

Clowse, Megan E. B., "Lupus Activity in Pregnancy," *Rheumatic Disease Clinics of North America* 33, no. 2 (2007): 237–v. https://www.ncbi.nlm.nih.gov/pmc/articles/PMC2745966/.

Clowse, Megan E. B., and Chad Grotegut, "Racial and Ethnic Disparities in the Pregnancies of Women with Systemic Lupus Erythematosus," *Arthritis Care Research* 68, no. 10 (October 2016): 1567–1572. https://doi.org/10.1002/acr.22847.

Clowse, Megan E. B., Margaret Jamison, Evan Myers, and Andra H. James, "A National Study of Medical Complications in SLE Pregnancies," *Arthritis and Rheumatism* 54, no. 9 (September 2006): P127.E1–127.E6, https://doi.org/10.1016/j.ajog.2008.03.012.

Cohn, Erica, dir. *Belly of the Beast* (Belly of the Beast LLC, Idle Wild Films, Independent Television Services & Black Public Media, 2020).

Collins, Jr., James W., Shou-Yien Wu, and Richard J. David, "Differing Intergenerational Birth Weights among the Descendants of US-Born and Foreign-Born Whites and African Americans in

Illinois," *American Journal of Epidemiology* 155, no. 3 (February 2002): 210–216. https://doi.org/10.1093/aje/155.3.210.

Colorado Department of Public Health and Environment, "Recommendations to Reduce Preterm Birth in Colorado," accessed June 10, 2022, https://cdphe.colorado.gov/sites/cdphe/files/PF_Preterm-BirthRecs.pdf.

"COVID-19 Vaccination Considerations for Obstetric–Gynecologic Care," American College of Obstetricians and Gynecologists, last updated June 3, 2022, https://www.acog.org/clinical/clinical-guidance/practice-advisory/articles/2020/12/covid-19-vaccination-considerations-for-obstetric-gynecologic-care.

Crouse Quinn, Sandra, Amelia Jamison, Ji An, Vicki S. Freimuth, Gregory R. Hancock, and Donald Musa, "Breaking Down the Monolith: Understanding Flu Vaccine Uptake among African Americans," *SSM—Population Health* 4 (2018): 25–36. https://doi.org/10.1016/j.ssmph.2017.11.003.

Cummings, Mike, "Numbers, Not Narratives, Remedy Misperceptions of the Racial Wealth Gap," Yale News, September 13, 2021, https://news.yale.edu/2021/09/13/numbers-not-narratives-remedy-misperceptions-racial-wealth-gap.

"Current Trends Infant Mortality—United States, 1992," *Morbidity and Mortality Weekly Report Weekly* 43, no. 49 (December 16, 1994): 905–909. https://www.cdc.gov/mmwr/preview/mmwrhtml/00033948.htm.

D'Ambrosio, Amanda, "Black Doctor Dies After Giving Birth, Underscoring Maternal Mortality Crisis," MedPage Today, November 2, 2020, https://www.medpagetoday.com/obgyn/pregnancy/89462.

———, "High-Quality Diet Cut Risk of Fetal Growth Restriction," MedPage Today, February 3, 2022, https://www.medpagetoday.com/meetingcoverage/smfm/97015.

David, Richard J., and James W. Collins, "Differing Birth Weight among Infants of U.S.-Born Blacks, African-Born Blacks, and U.S.-Born Whites," *New England Journal of Medicine* 337, no. 17 (1997): 1209–1214. https://doi.org/10.1056/NEJM199710233371706.

Debbink, Michelle P., Lynda G. Ugwu, William A. Grobman, Uma M. Reddy, Alan T. N. Tita, Yasser Y. El-Sayed, Ronald J. Wapner,

Dwight J. Rouse, George R. Saade, John M. Thorp Jr., Suneet P. Chauhan, Maged M. Costantine, Edward K. Chien, Brian M. Casey, Sindhu K. Srinivas, Geeta K. Swamy, and Hyagriv N. Simhan, "Racial and Ethnic Inequities in Cesarean Birth and Maternal Morbidity in a Low-Risk, Nulliparous Cohort," *Obstetrics & Gynecology* 139, no. 1 (January 2022): 73–82. https://doi.org/10.1097/AOG.0000000000004620.

"Delivery Method," March of Dimes, updated January 2022, https://www.marchofdimes.org/peristats/data?reg=99&top=8&stop=356&lev=1&slev=1&obj=1.

DePietro, Mary Ann, and Clarissa Stephens, "What Is the Average Baby Weight by Month?," *Medical News Today*, September 6, 2021, https://www.medicalnewstoday.com/articles/325630.

DeSisto, Carla L., Bailey Wallace, Regina M. Simeone, Kara Polen, Jean Y. Ko, Dana Meaney-Delman, and Sascha R. Ellington, "Risk for Stillbirth Among Women with and without COVID-19 at Delivery Hospitalization—United States, March 2020–September 2021," *Morbidity and Mortality Weekly Report* 70, no. 47 (November 26, 2021): 1640–1645. https://www.cdc.gov/mmwr/volumes/70/wr/mm7047e1.htm.

Devine, Patricia G., Patrick S. Forscher, Anthony J. Austin, and William T. L. Cox, "Long-term Reduction in Implicit Race Bias: A Prejudice Habit-Breaking Intervention," *Journal of Experimental Social Psychology* 48, no. 6 (November 2012): 1267–1278. https://doi.org/10.1016/j.jesp.2012.06.003.

Din-Dzietham, R., and I. Hertz-Picciotto, "Infant Mortality Difference between Whites and African Americans: The Effect of Maternal Education," *American Journal of Public Health* 88, no. 4 (1998): 651–656. https://doi.org/10.2105/AJPH.88.4.651.

Dockser Marcus, Amy, "Sperm Banks Struggle to Recruit Black Donors and Other Donors of Color," *Wall Street Journal*, February 26, 2022, https://www.wsj.com/articles/sperm-banks-struggle-to-recruit-black-donors-and-other-donors-of-color-11645887602.

Dominguez, Tyan Parker, Emily Ficklin Strong, Nancy Krieger, Matthew W. Gillman, and Janet W. Rich-Edwards, "Differences in the Self-Reported Racism Experiences of US-Born and Foreign-Born Black Pregnant Women," *Social Science & Medicine* 69, no. 2 (2009): 258–265. https://doi.org/10.1016/j.socscimed.2009.03.022.

Donnelly, Erin, and Stacy Jackman, "The Emotional Story Behind the World's Most Premature Baby: 'He Was Able to Show Us That He Was Bigger and Stronger Than We Expected,'" Yahoo!Life, February 23, 2022, https://www.yahoo.com/lifestyle/worlds-most-premature-baby-curtis-means-172139245.html.

Doula Medicaid Project, National Health Law Program, accessed April 25, 2022, https://healthlaw.org/doulamedicaidproject/.

Dr. Shalon's Maternal Action Project, accessed June 4, 2022, https://www.drshalonsmap.org/.

Dudley, Matthew Z., Rupali J. Limaye, Daniel A. Salmon, Saad B. Omer, Sean T. O'Leary, Mallory K. Ellingson, Christine I. Spina, Sarah E. Brewer, Robert A. Bednarczyk, Fauzia Malik, Paula M. Frew, and Allison T. Chamberlain, "Racial/Ethnic Disparities in Maternal Vaccine Knowledge, Attitudes, and Intentions," *Public Health Reports* 136, no. 6 (November–December 2021): 699–709. https://doi.org/10.1177/003335492x0974660.

Dugas, Carla, and Valori H. Slane, "Miscarriage," National Library of Medicine, last updated May 8, 2022, https://www.ncbi.nlm.nih.gov/books/NBK532992/.

Earth's Natural Touch, accessed June 6, 2022, https://earthsnaturaltouch.com/.

Echols, Hannah, "UAB Hospital Delivers Record-Breaking Premature Baby," Health & Medicine, University of Alabama News, November 10, 2021, https://www.uab.edu/news/health/item/12427-uab-hospital-delivers-record-breaking-premature-baby.

"Electronic Medical Records/Electronic Health Records (EMRs/EHRs)," Centers for Disease Control and Prevention, last updated

October 14, 2021, https://www.cdc.gov/nchs/fastats/electronic-medical-records.htm.

Eliason, Erica L., "Adoption of Medicaid Expansion is Associated with Lower Maternal Mortality," *Women's Health Issues* 30, no. 3 (May 2020): 147–152. https://doi.org/10.1016/j.whi.2020.01.005.

Ellen Boakye, Yaa Adoma Kwapong, Olufunmilayo Obisesan, S. Michelle Ogunwole, Allison G. Hays, Khurram Nasir, Roger S. Blumenthal, Pamela S. Douglas, Michael J. Blaha, Xiumei Hong, Andreea A. Creanga, Xiaobin Wang, Garima Sharma, "Nativity-Related Disparities in Preeclampsia and Cardiovascular Disease Risk Among a Racially Diverse Cohort of US Women," *JAMA Network Open* 4, no. 12 (2021): e2139564. https://doi.org/10.1001/jamanetworkopen.2021.39564.

Ellerbe, Calvina, "Racial Differences in Marital Outcomes among Unmarried Mothers: The Influence of Perceived Marital Benefits and Expectations," Fragile Families Working Paper no. WP18-03-FF, January 2018, https://fragilefamilies.princeton.edu/sites/fragilefamilies/files/wp18-03-ff.pdf.

Ellington, Sascha, Penelope Strid, Van T. Tong, Kate Woodworth, Romeo R. Galang, Laura D. Zambrano, John Nahabedian, Kayla Anderson, and Suzanne M. Gilboa, "Characteristics of Women of Reproductive Age with Laboratory-Confirmed SARS-CoV-2 Infection by Pregnancy Status—United States, January 22–June 7, 2020," *Morbidity and Mortality Weekly Report* 69, no. 25 (June 26, 2020): 769–775. https://www.cdc.gov/mmwr/volumes/69/wr/mm6925a1.htm.

Elo, Irma T., Zoua Vang, and Jennifer F. Culhane, "Variation in Birth Outcomes by Mother's Country of Birth Among Non-Hispanic Black Women in the United States," *Maternal and Child Health Journal* 18, no. 10 (2014): 2371–2381. https://doi.org/10.1007/s10995-014-1477-0.

Eltoukhi, Heba M., Monica N. Modi, Meredith Weston, Alicia Y. Armstrong, and Elizabeth A. Stewart, "The Health Disparities of Uterine Fibroids for African American Women: A Public Health Issue," *American Journal of Obstetrics and Gynecology* 210, no. 3 (March 2014): 194–199. http://doi.org/10.1016/j.ajog.2013.08.008.

Ely, Danielle M., and Anne K. Driscoll, "Infant Mortality in the United States, 2018: Data from the Period Linked Birth/Infant Death File," *National Vital Statistics Reports* 69, no. 7 (July 16, 2020), https://www.cdc.gov/nchs/data/nvsr/nvsr69/NVSR-69-7-508.pdf.

"Eradicating Polio," UNICEF, accessed June 11, 2022, https://www.unicef.org/immunization/polio.

"Extend Postpartum Medicaid Coverage," American College of Obstetricians and Gynecologists, accessed April 10, 2022, https://www.acog.org/advocacy/policy-priorities/extend-postpartum-medicaid-coverage.

"Fact Sheet: Biden–Harris Administration Announces Additional Actions in Response to Vice President Harris's Call to Action on Maternal Health," White House, April 13, 2022, https://www.whitehouse.gov/briefing-room/statements-releases/2022/04/13/fact-sheet-biden-harris-administration-announces-additional-actions-in-response-to-vice-president-harriss-call-to-action-on-maternal-health/.

"Fact Sheet: Vice President Kamala Harris Announces Call to Action to Reduce Maternal Mortality and Morbidity," White House, December 7, 2021, https://www.whitehouse.gov/briefing-room/statements-releases/2021/12/07/fact-sheet-vice-president-kamala-harris-announces-call-to-action-to-reduce-maternal-mortality-and-morbidity/.

Feldman, Candace H., Linda T. Hiraki, Jun Liu, Michael A. Fischer, Daniel H. Solomon, Graciela S. Alarcón, Wolfgang C. Winkelmayer, and Karen H. Costenbader, "Epidemiology and Sociodemographics of Systemic Lupus Erythematosus and Lupus Nephritis among U.S. Adults with Medicaid Coverage, 2000–2004," *Arthritis Rheumatism* 65, no. 3 (March 2013): 753–763. https://doi.org/10.1002/art.37795.

"Female Physicians Face Higher Rates of Infertility and Pregnancy Complications," *ASH Clinical News*, November 2021, https://ashpublications.org/ashclinicalnews/news/1426/Female-Physicians-Face-Higher-Rates-of-Infertility.

FitzGerald, Chloë, and Samia Hurst, "Implicit Bias in Healthcare Professionals: A Systematic Review," *BMC Medical Ethics*, no. 18 (2017): art. 19. https://doi.org/10.1186/s12910-017-0179-8.

Frias, Antonio E., Terry K. Morgan, Anne E. Evans, Juha Rasanen, Karen Y. Oh, Kent L. Thornburg, and Kevin L. Grove, "Maternal High-Fat Diet Disturbs Uteroplacental Hemodynamics and Increases the Frequency of Stillbirth in a Nonhuman Primate Model of Excess Nutrition," *Endocrinology* 152, no. 6 (June 1, 2011): 2456–2464, https://doi.org/10.1210/en.2010-1332.

Fu, Linda Y., Rachel Y. Moon, and Fern R. Hauck, "Bed Sharing among Black Infants and Sudden Infant Death Syndrome: Interactions with Other Known Risk Factors," *Prevention* 10, no. 6 (November 2010): 376–382. https://doi.org/10.1016/j.acap.2010.09.001.

Gawel, Richard, "Hispanic, Black Women Less Likely to Use Fertility Treatment Even with Insurance Coverage," Women's Health & OB/GYN, October 18, 2021, https://www.healio.com/news/womens-health-ob-gyn/20211018/hispanic-black-women-less-likely-to-use-fertility-treatment-even-with-insurance-coverage.

Geronimus, Arline T., Margaret T. Hicken, Danya Keene, and John Bound, "'Weathering' and Age Patterns of Allostatic Load Scores Among Blacks and Whites in the United States," *American Journal of Public Health* 96, no. 5 (May 2006): 826–833. https://doi.org/10.2105/AJPH.2004.060749.

Geronimus, Arline T., Margaret T. Hicken, Jay A. Pearson, Sarah J. Seashols, Kelly L. Brown, and Tracey Dawson Cruz, "Do US Black Women Experience Stress-Related Accelerated Biological Aging? A Novel Theory and First Population-Based Test of Black–White Differences in Telomere Length," *Human Nature* 21, no. 1 (March 2010): 19–38. https://doi.org/10.1007/s12110-010-9078-0.

"Gestational Hypertension and Preeclampsia," *ACOG Practice Bulletin*, no. 222 (June 2020), https://www.acog.org/clinical/clinical-guidance/practice-bulletin/articles/2020/06/gestational-hypertension-and-preeclampsia.

Ghosh, Gaurav, Jagteshwar Grewal, Tuija Männistö, Pauline Mendola, Zhen Chen, Yunlong Xie, and S. Katherine Laughon, "Racial/Ethnic Differences in Pregnancy-Related Hypertensive Disease in Nulliparous Women," *Ethnicity and Disease* 24, no. 3 (2014): 283–289. https://www.ncbi.nlm.nih.gov/pmc/articles/PMC4171100/.

Gibson, Bentley L., Philippe Rochat, Erin B. Tone, and Andrew S. Baron, "Sources of Implicit and Explicit Intergroup Race Bias among African-American Children and Young Adults," *PloS One* 12, no. 9 (September 2017): e0183015. https://doi.org/10.1371/journal.pone.0183015.

Giscombé, Cheryl L., and Marci Lobel, "Explaining Disproportionately High Rates of Adverse Birth Outcomes Among African Americans: The Impact of Stress, Racism, and Related Factors in Pregnancy," *Psychology Bulletin* 131, no. 5 (2005): 662–683. https://doi.org/10.1037/0033-2909.131.5.662.

Goldenberg, Robert L., Suzanne P. Cliver, Francis X. Mulvihill, Carol A. Hickey, Howard J. Hoffman, Lorraine V. Klerman, and Marilyn J. Johnson, "Medical, Psychosocial, and Behavioral Risk Factors Do Not Explain the Increased Risk for Low Birth Weight Among Black Women," *American Journal of Obstetrics and Gynecology* 175, no. 5 (November 1996): 1317–1324. https://doi.org/10.1016/s0002-9378(96)70048-0.

Goodnight, William H., and Roger B. Newman, "Optimal Nutrition for Improved Twin Pregnancy Outcome," *Obstetrics & Gynecology* 114, no. 5 (2009): 1121–1134. https://doi.org/10.1097/AOG.0b013e3181bb14c8.

Goodwin, Gerald F., "Black and White in Vietnam," *New York Times*, July 18, 2017, https://www.nytimes.com/2017/07/18/opinion/racism-vietnam-war.html.

Gramlich, John, "Black Imprisonment Rate in the U.S. Has Fallen by a Third Since 2006," Pew Research Center, May 6, 2020, https://www.pewresearch.org/fact-tank/2020/05/06/share-of-black-white-hispanic-americans-in-prison-2018-vs-2006/.

Grant, Jacqueline H., Catherine J. Vladutiu, and Tracy A. Manuck, "Racial Disparities in Delivery Gestational Age among Twin Pregnancies," *American Journal of Perinatology* 34, no. 11 (2017): 1065–1071. http://doi.org/10.1055/s-0037-1603764.

Green, Alexander R., Dana R. Carney, Daniel J. Pallin, Long H. Ngo, Kristal L. Raymond, Lisa I. Iezzoni, and Mahzarin R. Banaji,

"Implicit Bias among Physicians and its Prediction of Thrombolysis Decisions for Black and White Patients," *Journal of General Internal Medicine* 22, no. 9 (2007): 1231–1238. https://doi.org/10.1007/s11606-007-0258-5.

Green, Rochelle S., Brian Malig, Gayle C. Windham, Laura Fenster, Bart Ostro, and Shanna Swan, "Residential Exposure to Traffic and Spontaneous Abortion," *Environmental Health Perspectives* 117, no. 12 (December 2009): 1939–1944. http://doi.org/10.1289/ehp.0900943.

Green, Susan, "Violence Against Black Women—Many Types, Far-Reaching Effects," Institute for Women's Policy Research, July 13, 2017, https://iwpr.org/iwpr-issues/race-ethnicity-gender-and-economy/violence-against-black-women-many-types-far-reaching-effects/.

Greenwood, Brad N., Rachel R. Hardeman, Laura Huang, and Aaron Sojourner, "Patient Racial Concordance and Disparities in Birthing Mortality for Newborns," *Proceedings of the National Academy of Sciences* 117, no. 35 (2020): 21194–21200. https://doi.org/10.1073/pnas.1913405117.

Gregory, Elizabeth C.W., Claudia P. Valenzuela, and Donna L. Hoyert, "Fetal Mortality: United States, 2019," *National Vital Statistics Reports* 70, no. 11 (October 26, 2021), https://www.cdc.gov/nchs/data/nvsr/nvsr70/nvsr70-11.pdf.

Gregory, Kimberly D., Sherri Jackson, Lisa Korst, and Moshe Fridman, "Cesarean versus Vaginal Delivery: Whose Risks? Whose Benefits?," *American Journal Perinatology* 29, no. 1 (2012): 7–18. https://doi.org/10.1055/s-0031-1285829.

Grobman, William A., Madeline M. Rice, Uma M. Reddy, Alan T. N. Tita, Robert M. Silver, Gail Mallett, Kim Hill, Elizabeth A. Thom, Yasser Y. El-Sayed, Annette Perez-Delboy, Dwight J. Rouse, George R. Saade, Kim A. Boggess, Suneet P. Chauhan, Jay D. Iams, Edward K. Chien, Brian M. Casey, Ronald S. Gibbs, Sindhu K. Srinivas, Geeta K. Swamy, Hyagriv N. Simhan, and George A. Macones, "Labor Induction Versus Expectant Management in Low-Risk Nulliparous Women," *New England Journal of Medicine* 379 (2018): 513–523. https://doi.org/10.1056/NEJMoa1800566.

Grow, Elizabeth, "'How Dare You Adopt a White Baby?!' 'We Only Had the Desire to Become Parents': Couple Battling Male Factor Infertility Build Transracial Family through Adoption, Embryo Donations," Love What Matters, accessed June 11, 2022, https://www.lovewhatmatters.com/couple-battling-male-factor-infertility-build-transracial-family-through-adoption-embryo-donations/.

Gruber, Kenneth J., Susan H. Cupito, and Christina F. Dobson, "Impact of Doulas on Healthy Birth Outcomes," *Journal of Perinatal Education* 22, no. 1 (Winter 2013): 49. https://doi.org/10.1891/1058-1243.22.1.49.

Guidi, J., M. Lucente, N. Sonino, and G.A. Fava, "Allostatic Load and Its Impact on Health: A Systematic Review," *Psychotherapy and Psychosomatics* 90, no. 11 (2021): 11–27. https://doi.org/10.1159/000510696.

H.R.1318—Preventing Maternal Deaths Act of 2018, 115th Cong. (2017–2018), https://www.congress.gov/bill/115th-congress/house-bill/1318/text.

H.R.4387—Maternal Health Quality Improvement Act of 2021, 117th Cong. (2021–2022), https://www.congress.gov/bill/117th-congress/house-bill/4387.

H.R.959–Black Maternal Health Momnibus Act of 2021, 117th Cong. (2021–2022), https://www.congress.gov/bill/117th-congress/house-bill/959.

Halasa, Natasha B., Samantha M. Olson, Mary A. Staat, Margaret M. Newhams, Ashley M. Price, Julie A. Boom, Leila C. Sahni, Melissa A. Cameron, Pia S. Pannaraj, Katherine E. Bline, Samina S. Bhumbra, Tamara T. Bradford, Kathleen Chiotos, Bria M. Coates, Melissa L. Cullimore, Natalie Z. Cvijanovich, Heidi R. Flori, Shira J. Gertz, Sabrina M. Heidemann, Charlotte V. Hobbs, Janet R. Hume, Katherine Irby, Satoshi Kamidani, Michele Kong, Emily R. Levy, Elizabeth H. Mack, Aline B. Maddux, Kelly N. Michelson, Ryan A. Nofziger, Jennifer E. Schuster, Stephanie P. Schwartz, Laura Smallcomb, Keiko M. Tarquinio, Tracie C. Walker, Matt S. Zinter, Suzanne M. Gilboa, Kara N. Polen, Angela P. Campbell, Adrienne G. Randolph, and Manish M. Patel, "Effectiveness of Maternal Vaccination with mRNA COVID-19 Vaccine During Pregnancy Against COVID-19–Associated Hospitalization in Infants Aged <6 Months—17 States, July 2021–January 2022," *Morbidity and Mortality Weekly Report* 71, no. 7 (February 18, 2022): 264–270. https://www.cdc.gov/mmwr/volumes/71/wr/mm7107e3.htm.

Handal-Orefice, Roxane C., Melissa McHale, Alexander M. Friedman, Joseph A. Politch, and Wendy Kuohung, "Impact of Race Versus Ethnicity on Infertility Diagnosis between Black American, Haitian, African, and White American Women Seeking Infertility Care: A Retrospective Review," *F&S Reports* 3, no. 2 Suppl. (May 2022): 22–28. https://doi.org/10.1016/j.xfre.2021.11.003.

Hasbini, Yasmin G., Gregory Goyert, Adi L. Tarca, Madhurima Keerthy, Theodore Jones, Lisa Thiel, Pooja M. Green, Youssef Youssef, Courtney Townsel, Shyla Vengalil, Paige Paladino, Amy Wright, Mariam Ayyash, Gayathri Vadlamudi, Marta Szymanska, Sonia Sajja, Grace Sterenberg, Michael Baracy Jr., Karlee Grace, Kaitlyn Houston, Jessica Norman, Dereje W. Gudicha, Robert J. Sokol, Ray Bahado-Singh, and Sonia S. Hassan, "COVID-19 is Associated with Early Emergence of Preeclampsia: Results from a Large Regional Collaborative," *American Journal of Obstetrics and Gynecology* 226, no. 1 (2022), S594–S595. https://doi.org/10.1016/j.ajog.2021.11.980.

Haskell, Rob, "Serena Williams on Motherhood, Miscarriage and Making Her Comeback," *Vogue*, January 10, 2018, https://www.vogue.com/article/serena-williams-vogue-cover-interview-february-2018.

"Haywood Brown, MD Becomes 68th President of ACOG," Duke Obstetrics & Gynecology, May 9, 2017, https://obgyn.duke.edu/news/haywood-brown-md-becomes-68th-president-acog.

"Health Literacy Universal Precautions Toolkit, 2nd Edition," Agency for Healthcare Research and Quality, last updated September 2020, https://www.ahrq.gov/health-literacy/improve/precautions/tool2b.html.

Hemez, Paul, and Chanell Washington, "Percentage and Number of Children Living with Two Parents Has Dropped Since 1968," United States Census Bureau, April 12, 2021, https://www.census.gov/library/stories/2021/04/number

-of-children-living-only-with-their-mothers-has-doubled-in-past-50-years.html.

Hogue, Carol J. R., Corette B. Parker, Marian Willinger, Jeff R. Temple, Carla M. Bann, Robert M. Silver, Donald J. Dudley, Matthew A. Koch, Donald R. Coustan, Barbara J. Stoll, Uma M. Reddy, Michael W. Varner, George R. Saade, Deborah Conway, and Robert L. Goldenberg, "A Population-Based Case-Control Study of Stillbirth: The Relationship of Significant Life Events to the Racial Disparity for African Americans," *American Journal of Epidemiology* 177, no. 8 (2013): 755–767. https://doi.org/10.1093/aje/kws381.

Holgash, Kayla, and Martha Heberlein, "Physician Acceptance of New Medicaid Patients: What Matters and What Doesn't," *Health Affairs*, April 10, 2019, https://doi.org/10.1377/forefront.20190401.678690.

Holmes, Laurens, Leah O'Neill, Hikma Elmi, Chinaka Chinacherem, Camillia Comeaux, Lavisha Pelaez, Kirk W. Dabney, Olumuyiwa Akinola, and Michael Enwere, "Implication of Vaginal and Cesarean Section Delivery Method in Black–White Differentials in Infant Mortality in the United States: Linked Birth/Infant Death Records, 2007–2016," *International Journal of Environmental Research and Public Health* 17, no. 9 (May 2020): 3146. https://doi.org/10.3390/ijerph17093146.

"Homelessness and Racial Disparities," National Alliance to End Homelessness, updated October 2020, https://endhomelessness.org/homelessness-in-america/what-causes-homelessness/inequality/.

Howell, Elizabeth A., "Reducing Disparities in Severe Maternal Morbidity and Mortality," *Clinical Obstetrics and Gynecology* 61, no. 2 (June 2018): 387–399. http://doi.org/10.1097/GRF.0000000000000349.

Hoyert, Donna L., "Maternal Mortality Rates in the United States, 2020," National Center for Health Statistics, Centers for Disease Control and Prevention, last updated February 23, 2022, https://www.cdc.gov/nchs/data/hestat/maternal-mortality/2020/maternal-mortality-rates-2020.htm.

Huesch, Marco, and Jason N. Doctor, "Factors Associated with Increased Cesarean Section Risk Among African American Women: Evidence from California, 2010," *American Journal of Public Health* 105, no. 5 (May 2015): 956. https://doi.org/10.2105/AJPH.2014.302381.

Hughes, Karen, Mark A. Bellis, Katherine A. Hardcastle, Dinesh Sethi, Alexander Butchart, Christopher Mikton, Lisa Jones, Michael P. Dunne, "The Effect of Multiple Adverse Childhood Experiences on Health: A Systematic Review and Meta-analysis," *Lancet Public Health* 2, no. 8 (2017): e356–366. https://doi.org/10.1016/S2468-2667(17)30118-4.

Hui, Kayla, "How One App Is Helping Black Women Find Culturally Competent Care," very well health, January 6, 2022, https://www.verywellhealth.com/health-in-her-hue-app-5214764.

Ickovics, Jeannette R., Trace S. Kershaw, Claire Westdahl, Urania Magriples, Zohar Massey, Heather Reynolds, and Sharon Schindler Rising, "Group Prenatal Care and Perinatal Outcomes: A Randomized Controlled Trial," *Obstetrics & Gynecology* 110, no. 2.1 (August 2007): 330–339. https://doi.org/10.1097/01.AOG.0000275284.24298.23.

"Infant Mortality," Centers for Disease Control and Prevention, last updated June 22, 2022, https://www.cdc.gov/reproductivehealth/maternalinfanthealth/infantmortality.htm.

"Infant Mortality and African Americans," U.S. Department of Health and Human Services, Office of Minority Health, last updated July 8, 2021. https://minorityhealth.hhs.gov/omh/browse.aspx?lvl=4&lvlid=23.

"Infertility FAQs," Centers for Disease Control and Prevention, last updated March 1, 2022, https://www.cdc.gov/reproductivehealth/infertility/index.htm.

Jacob, Kevin, and Jacob E. Hoerter, *Caput Succedaneum* (StatPearls Publishing, 2022). https://www.ncbi.nlm.nih.gov/books/NBK574534/.

Jameson, J. Larry, and Kevin B. Mahoney, Communication from the Dean to Faculty, Students, and Staff and UPHS Leadership, "Appointment of Elizabeth A. Howell, MD, MPP, as Chair of the Department of Obstetrics and Gynecology," Perelmann

School of Medicine, University of Pennsylvania, May 12, 2020, https://www.med.upenn.edu/evpdeancommunications/2020-05-12-210.html.

"January 3, 1938: Franklin Roosevelt Founds March of Dimes," This Day in History, History.com, last modified January 2, 2020, https://www.history.com/this-day-in-history/franklin-roosevelt-founds-march-of-dimes.

Jenerette, Coretta M., and Cheryl Brewer, "Health-Related Stigma in Young Adults with Sickle Cell Disease," *Journal of the National Medical Association* 102, no. 11 (2010): 1050–1055. https://doi.org/10.1016/s0027-9684(15)30732-x.

Jercich, Kat, "U.S. Clinicians Spend 50% More Time in EHR than Those in Other Countries," HealthcareITNews, December 17, 2020, https://www.healthcareitnews.com/news/us-clinicians-spend-50-more-time-ehr-those-other-countries.

Jin, Jill, "Babies with Low Birth Weight," *JAMA* 313, no. 4 (2015): 432. https://doi.org/10.1001/jama.2014.3698.

The JJ WAY®: Community-Based Maternity Center Final Evaluation Report, Visionary Vanguard Group, 2017, https://secureserver cdn.net/198.71.233.72/qj7.106.myftpupload.com/wp-content/uploads/2022/03/The-JJ-Way®-Community-based-Maternity-Center-Evaluation-Report-2017-1.pdf.

Johnson, Rucker C., and Robert F. Schoeni, "The Influence of Early-Life Events on Human Capital, Health Status, and Labor Market Outcomes Over the Life Course," National Poverty Center Working Paper Series, Paper No. 07-05, February 2007, http://npc.umich.edu/publications/u/working_paper05-07.pdf.

Joyner, Brandi L., Rosalind P. Oden, Taiwo I. Ajao, and Rachel Y. Moon, "Where Should My Baby Sleep: A Qualitative Study of African American Infant Sleep Location Decisions," *Journal of the National Medical Association* 102, no. 10 (2010): 881–889. https://doi.org/10.1016/S0027-9684(15)30706-9.

Kalmoe, Molly C., Matthew B. Chapman, Jessica A. Gold, and Andrea M. Giedinghagen, "Physician Suicide: A Call to Action," *Missouri Medicine* 116, no. 3 (2019): 211–216. https://www.ncbi.nlm.nih.gov/pmc/articles/PMC6690303/.

Kane, Leslie, "'Death by 1000 Cuts': Medscape National Physician Burnout & Suicide Report 2021," Medscape, January 22, 2021, https://www.medscape.com/slideshow/2021-lifestyle-burnout-6013456.

Kasehagen, Laurin, Paul Byers, Kathryn Taylor, Theresa Kittle, Christine Roberts, Charlene Collier, Britney Rust, Jessica N. Ricaldi, Jamilla Green, Lauren B. Zapata, Jennifer Beauregard, and Thomas Dobbs, "COVID-19–Associated Deaths after SARS-CoV-2 Infection During Pregnancy—Mississippi, March 1, 2020–October 6, 2021," *Morbidity and Mortality Weekly Report* 70, no. 47 (November 26, 2021): 1646–1648. https://www.cdc.gov/mmwr/volumes/70/wr/mm7047e2.htm.

Keag, Oonagh E., Jane E. Norman, and Sarah J. Stock, "Long-term Risks and Benefits Associated with Cesarean Delivery for Mother, Baby, and Subsequent Pregnancies: Systematic Review and Meta-analysis," *PLoS medicine* 15, no. 1 (2018): e1002494. https://doi.org/10.1371/journal.pmed.1002494.

Khoury, Janette, Tore Henriksen, Bjørn Christophersen, and Serena Tonstad, "Effect of a Cholesterol-Lowering Diet on Maternal, Cord, and Neonatal Lipids, and Pregnancy Outcome: A Randomized Clinical Trial," *American Journal of Obstetrics and Gynecology* 193, no. 4 (October 2005): 1292–1301. http://doi.org/10.1016/j.ajog.2005.05.016.

Kilich, Eliz, Sara Dada, and Mark R. Francis, "Factors that Influence Vaccination Decision-Making among Pregnant Women: A Systematic Review and Meta-analysis," *PLOS One*, July 9, 2020, https://doi.org/10.1371/journal.pone.0234827.

"Kira Johnson, Cedars-Sinai Los Angeles," Consumer Watchdog, accessed May 30, 2022, https://www.consumerwatchdog.org/patient-safety/kira-johnson-cedars-sinai-los-angeles.

Kochanek, Kenneth D., Jiaquan Xu, and Elizabeth Arias, "Mortality in the United States, 2019," *NCHS Data Brief*, no. 395 (December 2020), fig. 5 data table, https://www.cdc.gov/nchs/data/databriefs/db395-H.pdf.

Kozhimannil, Katy B., Peiyin Hung, Carrie Henning-Smith, Michelle M. Casey, and Shailendra Prasad, "Association between Loss of Hospital-Based Obstetric Services and Birth Outcomes in Rural

Counties in the United States," *JAMA* 319, no. 12 (2018): 1239–1247. https://doi.org/10.1001/jama.2018.1830.

Kozhimannil, Katy B., Rachel R. Hardeman, Fernando Alarid-Escudero, Carrie A. Vogelsang, Cori Blauer-Peterson, and Elizabeth A. Howell, "Modeling the Cost-Effectiveness of Doula Care Associated with Reductions in Preterm Birth and Cesarean Delivery," *Birth* 43, no. 1 (March 2016): 20–27. http://doi.org/10.1111/birt.12218.

Kreiger, Nancy, "Discrimination and Health Inequities," *International Journal of Health Services* 44, no. 4 (2014): 643–710. https://doi.org/0.2190/HS.44.4.b.

La Puma, John, "What Is Culinary Medicine and What Does It Do?," *Population Health Management* 19, no. 1 (February 2016): 1–3. https://doi.org/10.1089/pop.2015.0003.

Lanzkron, Sophie, C. Patrick Carroll, and Carlton Haywood, Jr., Mortality Rates and Age at Death from Sickle Cell Disease: U.S., 1979–2005," *Public Health Reports* 128, no. 2 (March–April 2013): 110–116. https://doi.org/10.1177/003335491312800206.

Lassi, Zohra S., and Zulfiqar A. Bhutta, "Community-Based Intervention Packages for Reducing Maternal and Neonatal Morbidity and Mortality and Improving Neonatal Outcomes," *Cochrane Database of Systematic Reviews*, no. 4 (2016), https://doi.org/10.1002/14651858.CD007754.pub3.

Lassi, Zohra S., Jai K. Das, Rehana A. Salam, and Zulfiqar A. Bhutta, "Evidence from Community Level Inputs to Improve Quality of Care for Maternal and Newborn Health: Interventions and Findings, *Reproductive Health* 11 (2014): art. S2. https://doi.org/10.1186/1742-4755-11-S2-S2.

Lassi, Zohra S., Zahra A. Padhani, Amna Rabbani, Fahad Rind, Rehana A. Salam, and Zulfiqar A. Bhutta, "Effects of Nutritional Interventions During Pregnancy on Birth, Child Health and Development Outcomes: A Systematic Review of Evidence from Low- and Middle-Income Countries," *Campbell Systematic Reviews* 17, no. 2 (2021): e1150. https://doi.org/10.1002/cl2.1150.

Laumbach, Robert, Qingyu Meng, and Howard Kipen, "What Can Individuals Do to Reduce Personal Health Risks from Air

Pollution?," *Journal of Thoracic Disease* 7, no. 1 (January 2015): 96–107. http://doi.org/10.3978/j.issn.2072-1439.2014.12.21.

Lee, Eunju, Susan D. Mitchell-Herzfeld, Ann A. Lowenfels, Rose Greene, Vajeera Dorabawila, and Kimberly A. DuMont, "Reducing Low Birth Weight Through Home Visitation: A Randomized Controlled Trial," *American Journal of Preventive Medicine* 36, no. 2 (2009): 154–160. https://doi.org/10.1016/j.amepre.2008.09.029.

Leung, Anna S., Eleanor K. Leung, and Richard H. Paul, "Uterine Rupture after Previous Cesarean Delivery: Maternal and Fetal Consequences," *American Journal of Obstetrics and Gynecology* 69, no. 4 (October 1993): 945–950, https://doi.org/10.1016/0002-9378(93)90032-E.

Livingston, Gretchen, and Anna Brown, "Trends and Patterns in Intermarriage," Pew Research Center, May 28, 2017, https://www.pewresearch.org/social-trends/2017/05/18/1-trends-and-patterns-in-intermarriage/.

"Low Birthweight," March of Dimes, last updated June 2021, https://www.marchofdimes.org/complications/low-birthweight.aspx.

Luke, Barbara, Morton B. Brown, Ruta Misiunas, Elaine Anderson, Clark Nugent, Cosmas van de Ven, Barbara Burpee, and Shirley Gogliotti, "Specialized Prenatal Care and Maternal and Infant Outcomes in Twin Pregnancy," *American Journal Obstetrics and Gynecology* 189, no. 4 (October 2003): 934–938. https://doi.org/10.1067/s0002-9378(03)01054-8.

Lydon-Rochelle, Mona, Victoria L. Holt, Thomas R. Easterling, and Diane P. Martin, "Risk of Uterine Rupture during Labor among Women with a Prior Cesarean Delivery," New England Journal of Medicine, no. 345 (July 2001): 3–8. https://doi.org/10.1056/NEJM200107053450101.

MacDorman, Marian F., Marie Thoma, Eugene Declcerq, and Elizabeth A. Howell, "Racial and Ethnic Disparities in Maternal Mortality in the United States Using Enhanced Vital Records, 2016–2017," *American Journal of Public Health* 111, no. 9 (2021): 1673–1681. https://doi.org/10.2105/AJPH.2021.306375.

"Management of Stillbirth," *Obstetric Care Consensus*, no. 10, March 2020, https://www.acog.org/clinical/clinical-guidance/obstetric-care-consensus/articles/2020/03/management-of-stillbirth.

Manuck, Tracy A., "Racial and Ethnic Differences in Preterm Birth: A Complex, Multifactorial Problem," *Seminars in Perinatology* 48, no. 8 (December 2017): 511–518. https://doi.org/10.1053/j.semperi.2017.08.010.

Marsa, Linda, "Labor Pains: The OB-GYN Shortage," Association of American Medical Colleges, November 15, 2018, https://www.aamc.org/news-insights/labor-pains-ob-gyn-shortage.

Martin, Joyce A., Brady E. Hamilton, and Michelle J.K. Osterman, "Births in the United States, *NCHS Data Brief*, no. 418 (September 2021), https://www.cdc.gov/nchs/data/databriefs/db418.pdf.

Martin, Joyce A., and Michelle J. K. Osterman, "Describing the Increase in Preterm Births in the United States, 2014–2016," *NCHS Data Brief*, no. 312 (June 2018), https://www.cdc.gov/nchs/data/databriefs/db312.pdf.

———, "Exploring the Decline in the Singleton Preterm Birth Rate in the United States, 2019–2022," *NCHS Data Brief*, no. 430 (January 2022), https://www.cdc.gov/nchs/data/databriefs/db430.pdf.

Martin, Joyce A., and Melissa M. Park, "Trends in Twin and Triplet Births: 1980–97," *National Vital Statistics Reports* 47, no. 24 (1999). https://www.cdc.gov/nchs/data/nvsr/nvsr47/nvs47_24.pdf.

Martin, Nina, and Renee Montagne, "Black Mothers Keep Dying After Giving Birth. Shalon Irving's Story Explains Why," NPR, December 7, 2017, https://www.npr.org/2017/12/07/568948782/black-mothers-keep-dying-after-giving-birth-shalon-irvings-story-explains-why.

"Maternal and Infant Characteristics Among Women with Confirmed or Presumed Cases of Coronavirus Disease (COVID-19) During Pregnancy," Centers for Disease Control and Prevention, last updated May 14, 2022, https://www.cdc.gov/nchs/covid19/technical-linkage.htm.

"Maternal Mortality—United States, 1982–1996," *Morbidity and Mortality Weekly Report* 47, no. 34 (September 4, 1998): 705–707.

https://www.cdc.gov/mmwr/preview/mmwrhtml/00054602. htm.

McCarther, Noria, Emily E. Daggett, Manesha Putra, "Racial Disparities in Severe Maternal Morbidity during Delivery Admission for People with Sickle Cell Anemia," *American Journal of Obstetrics and Gynecology* 226, no. 1 (2022): S673, https://doi.org/10.1016/j.ajog.2021.11.1111.

McEwen, Bruce S., and E. Stellar, "Stress and the Individual: Mechanisms Leading to Disease," *Archives of Internal Medicine* 153, no. 18 (September 1993): 2093–2101. https://doi.org/10.1001/archinte.1993.00410180039004.

McFarling, Usha Lee, "For Black Women, the Isolation of Infertility is Compounded by Barriers to Treatment," Stat, October 14, 2020, https://www.statnews.com/2020/10/14/for-black-women-isolation-of-infertility-compounded-by-barriers-to-treatment/.

McGrady, Gene A., John F. C. Sung, Diane L. Rowley, and Carol J. R. Hogue, "Preterm Delivery and Low Birth Weight Among First-Born Infants of Black and White College Graduates," *American Journal of Epidemiology* 136, no. 3 (August 1992): 266–276. https://doi.org/10.1093/oxfordjournals.aje.a116492.

Menacker, Fay, and Brady E. Hamilton, "Recent Trends in Cesarean Delivery in the United States," *NCHS Data Brief*, no. 35 (March 2010), https://www.cdc.gov/nchs/data/databriefs/db35.pdf.

"Mental Health Care Health Professional Shortage Areas (HPSAs)," Kaiser Family Foundation, last updated September 30, 2021, https://www.kff.org/other/state-indicator/mental-health-care-health-professional-shortage-areas-hpsas/.

Merino, Yesenia, Leslie Adams, and William J. Hall, "Implicit Bias and Mental Health Professionals: Priorities and Directions for Research," *Psychiatric Services* 69, no. 6 (2018): 723–725. https://doi.org/10.1176/appi.ps.201700294.

Minhas, Anum S., Xiumei Hong, Guoying Wang, Dong Keun Rhee, Tiange Liu, Mingyu Zhang, Erin D. Michos, Xiaobin Wang and Noel T. Mueller, "Mediterranean-Style Diet and Risk of Preeclampsia by Race in the Boston Birth Cohort" *Journal of the*

American Heart Association 11, no. 9 (2022): e022589. https://doi.org/10.1161/JAHA.121.022589.

"Momnibus," Black Maternal Health Caucus, accessed June 8, 2022, https://blackmaternalhealthcaucus-underwood.house.gov/Momnibus.

Mossburg, Cheri, and Taylor Romine, "Widower of Black Woman Who Died Hours after Childbirth Files Civil Rights Lawsuit against Cedars-Sinai," CNN, May 6, 2022, https://www.cnn.com/2022/05/06/us/california-civil-rights-lawsuit-cedars-sinai/index.html.

Motro, Daphna, Jonathan B. Evans, Aleksander P.J. Ellis, and Lehman Benson III, "The 'Angry Black Woman' Stereotype at Work," *Harvard Business Review*, January 31, 2022, https://hbr.org/2022/01/the-angry-black-woman-stereotype-at-work.

Mukherjee, Soumyadeep, Mary Jo Trepka, Dudith Pierre-Victor, Raed Bahelah, and Tenesha Avent, "Racial/Ethnic Disparities in Antenatal Depression in the United States: A Systematic Review," *Maternal and Child Health Journal* 20, no. 9 (September 2016): 1780–1797. https://doi.org/10.1007/s10995-016-1989-x.

Mukherjee, Sudeshna, Digna R. Velez Edwards, Donna D. Baird, David A. Savitz, and Katherine E. Hartmann, "Risk of Miscarriage Among Black Women and White Women in a US Prospective Cohort Study," *American Journal of Epidemiology* 177, no. 11 (June 2013): 1271–1278. https://doi.org/10.1093/aje/kws393.

"Multifetal Gestations Twin Triplet and Higher-Order Multifetal Pregnancies," *ACOG Practice Bulletin*, no. 231 (June 2021), https://www.acog.org/clinical/clinical-guidance/practice-bulletin/articles/2021/06/multifetal-gestations-twin-triplet-and-higher-order-multifetal-pregnancies.

Naftulin, Julia, "Inside the Hidden Campaign to Forcibly Sterilize Thousands of Inmates in California Women's Prisons," *Insider*, November 24, 2020, https://www.insider.com/inside-forced-sterilizations-california-womens-prisons-documentary-2020-11.

Ncube, Colette N., Daniel A. Enquobahrieb, Steven M. Alberta, Amy L. Herricka, and Jessica G. Burkea, "Association of Neighborhood Context with Offspring Risk of Preterm Birth and Low

Birthweight: A Systematic Review and Meta-Analysis of Population-Based Studies," *Social Science & Medicine* 153 (March 2016): 156–164. https://doi.org/10.1016/j.socscimed.2016.02.014.

Ndumele, Chima D., Michael S. Cohen, and Paul D. Cleary, "Association of State Access Standards with Accessibility to Specialists for Medicaid Managed Care Enrollees," *JAMA Internal Medicine* 177, no. 10 (2017): 1445–1451. https://jamanetwork.com/journals/jamainternalmedicine/fullarticle/2648744.

Nelson, David B., and Catherine Y. Spong, "Initiatives to Reduce Cesarean Delivery Rates for Low-Risk First Births," *JAMA* 325, no. 16 (2021): 1616–1617. https:/doi.org/10.1001/jama.2021.0084.

Nelson, Hannah, "OBGYNs Face Challenges When Providing Care to Medicaid Members," Healthpayer Intelligence, March 4, 2021, https://healthpayerintelligence.com/news/obgyns-face-challenges-when-providing-care-to-medicaid-members.

New Haven Early Start, Community Foundation for Greater New Haven, accessed June 13, 2022, https://www.cfgnh.org/leading-on-issues/healthy-families/new-haven-healthy-start.

New York City Department of Health and Mental Hygiene, "Severe Maternal Morbidity: New York City, 2008–2012," City of New York, 2016, https://www1.nyc.gov/assets/doh/downloads/pdf/data/maternal-morbidity-report-08-12.pdf.

Nguyen, Thu T., Nikki Adams, Dina Huang, M. Maria Glymour, Amani M. Allen, and Quynh C. Nguyen, "The Association Between State-Level Racial Attitudes Assessed from Twitter Data and Adverse Birth Outcomes: Observational Study," *JMIR Public Health Surveillance* 6, no. 3 (July 2020): e17103, https://doi.org/10.2196/17103.

Norbeck, Jane S., Jeanne F. DeJoseph, Renée T. Smith, "A Randomized Trial of an Empirically Derived Social Support Intervention to Prevent Low Birthweight among African American Women," *Social Science & Medicine* 43, no. 6 (1996): 947–954. https://doi.org/10.1016/0277-9536(96)00003-2.

O'Hare, Tom, and Francis Creed, "Life Events and Miscarriage," *British Journal of Psychiatry* 167, no. 6 (January 1995): 799–805. https://doi.org/10.1192/bjp.167.6.799.

Olds, David L., JoAnn Robinson, Lisa Pettitt, Dennis W. Luckey, John Holmberg, Rosanna K. Ng, Kathy Isacks, Karen Sheff, and Charles R. Henderson, Jr., "Effects of Home Visits by Paraprofessionals and by Nurses: Age 4 Follow-up Results of a Randomized Trial," *Pediatrics* 114, no. 6 (2004): 1560–1568. https://doi.org/10.1542/peds.2004-0961.

"Optimizing Postpartum Care," *Committee Opinion*, no. 736 (May 2018), https://www.acog.org/clinical/clinical-guidance/committee-opinion/articles/2018/05/optimizing-postpartum-care.

Oregon Health & Science University. "How High-Fat Diet During Pregnancy Increases Risk of Stillbirth," ScienceDaily, June 3, 2011, https://www.sciencedaily.com/releases/2011/06/110602153036.htm.

Osterman, Michelle J. K., Brady E. Hamilton, Joyce A. Martin, Anne K. Driscoll, and Claudia P. Valenzuela, "Births: Final Data for 2020," *National Vital Statistics Reports* 70, no. 17 (February 2020), https://www.cdc.gov/nchs/data/nvsr/nvsr70/nvsr70-17.pdf.

Ota, Erika, Katharina da Silva Lopes, Philippa Middleton, Vicki Flenady, Windy M.V. Wariki, Md. Obaidur Rahman, Ruoyan Tobe-Gai, and Rintaro Mori, "Antenatal Interventions for Preventing Stillbirth, Fetal Loss and Perinatal Death: An Overview of Cochrane Systematic Reviews," *Cochrane Database of Systematic Reviews*, no. 12 (2020), https://doi.org/10.1002/14651858.CD009599.pub2.

Ou, Christine H., and Wendy A. Hall, "Anger in the Context of Postnatal Depression: An Integrative Review," *Birth* 45, no. 4 (December 2018): 336–346. https://doi.org/10.1111/birt.12356.

"Our Impact," 4 Kira 4 Moms, accessed May 30, 2022, https://4kira4moms.com/who-are-we/.

"Our Story," Nurturely, accessed June 5, 2022, https://nurturely.org/mission/.

"Over One-Third of Americans Live in Areas Lacking Mental Health Professionals," USA Facts, last updated July 14, 2021, https://usafacts.org/articles/over-one-third-of-americans-live-in-areas-lacking-mental-health-professionals/.

Pallotto, Eugenia K., James W. Collins, Jr., and Richard J. David, "Enigma of Maternal Race and Infant Birth Weight: A Population-Based Study of US-Born Black and Caribbean-Born Black Women," *American Journal of Epidemiology* 151, no. 11 (June 2000): 1080–1085. https://doi.org/10.1093/oxfordjournals.aje.a010151.

Papageorghiou, Aris T., Philippe Deruelle, Robert B. Gunier, Stephen Rauch, Perla K. García-May, Mohak Mhatre, Mustapha Ado Usman, Sherief Abd-Elsalam, Saturday Etuk, Lavone E. Simmons, Raffaele Napolitano, Sonia Deantoni, Becky Liu, Federico Prefumo, Valeria Savasi, Marynéa Silva do Vale, Eric Baafi, Ghulam Zainab, Ricardo Nieto, Nerea Maiz, Muhammad Baffah Aminu, Jorge Arturo Cardona-Perez, Rachel Craik, Adele Winsey, Gabriela Tavchioska, Babagana Bako, Daniel Oros, Albertina Rego, Anne Caroline Benski, Fatimah Hassan-Hanga, Mónica Savorani, Francesca Giuliani, Loïc Sentilhes, Milagros Risso, Ken Takahashi, Carmen Vecchiarelli, Satoru Ikenoue, Ramachandran Thiruvengadam, Constanza P. Soto Conti, Enrico Ferrazzi, Irene Cetin, Vincent Bizor Nachinab, Ernawati Ernawati, Eduardo A. Duro, Alexey Kholin, Michelle L. Firlit, Sarah Rae Easter, Joanna Sichitiu, Abimbola Bowale, Roberto Casale, Rosa Maria Cerbo, Paolo Ivo Cavoretto, Brenda Eskenazi, Jim G. Thornton, Zulfiqar A. Bhutta, Stephen H. Kennedy, José Villar, "Preeclampsia and COVID-19: Results from the INTERCOVID Prospective Longitudinal Study," *American Journal of Obstetrics and Gynecology* 225, no. 3 (2021): P289.E1–P289.E17. https://doi.org/10.1016/j.ajog.2021.05.014.

Parker, Antay L., Lydia L. Forsythe, and Ingrid K. Kohlmorgen, "TeamSTEPPS®: An Evidence-Based Approach to Reduce Clinical Errors Threatening Safety in Outpatient Settings: An Integrative Review," *Journal of Healthcare Risk Management* 38, no. 4 (April 2019): 19–31. https://doi.org/10.1002/jhrm.21352.

Pérez, Miriam Zoila, "How Racism Harms Pregnant Women—and What Can Help," Filmed 2016, TED video. https://www.ted.com/talks/miriam_zoila_perez_how_racism_harms_pregnant_women_and_what_can_help/transcript.

Perl, Sivan Haia, Atara Uzan-Yulzari, Hodaya Klainer, Liron Asis-
    kovich, Michal Youngster, Ehud Rinott, and Ilan Young-
    ster, "SARS-CoV-2–Specific Antibodies in Breast Milk after
    COVID-19 Vaccination of Breastfeeding Women," *JAMA*
    325, no. 19 (2021): 2013–2014. https://doi.org/10.1001/
    jama.2021.5782.

Petersen, Emily E., Nicole L. Davis, David Goodman, Shanna Cox, Nikki
    Mayes; Emily Johnston, Carla Syverson, Kristi Seed, Carrie K.
    Shapiro-Mendoza, William M. Callaghan, and Wanda Barfield,
    "Vital Signs: Pregnancy-Related Deaths, United States, 2011–
    2015, and Strategies for Prevention, 13 States, 2013–2017,"
    Morbidity and Mortality Weekly Report 68, no. 18 (May 10,
    2019): 423–429. https://www.cdc.gov/mmwr/volumes/68/wr/
    mm6818e1.htm.

Pifer, Rebecca, "Black Women Disproportionately Concentrated in
    Low-Wage, Hazardous Healthcare Jobs, Study Finds," Health-
    careDive, February 8, 2022, https://www.healthcaredive.
    com/news/black-women-disproportionately-concentrated-
    low-wage-hazardous-health-jobs/618471/.

Pison, Gilles, "Nearly Half of the World's Twins are Born in Africa,"
    Population et sociétés, no. 360 (September 2000): 1–4. https://
    www.ined.fr/fichier/s_rubrique/18789/publi_pdf2_pop_and_
    soc_english_360.en.pdf.

Pollock, Elizabeth A., Keith P. Gennuso, Marjory L. Givens, and David
    Kindig, "Trends in Infants Born at Low Birthweight and Dispar-
    ities by Maternal Race and Education from 2003 to 2018 in the
    United States," *BMC Public Health*, no. 21 (2021): art. 1117.
    https://doi.org/10.1186/s12889-021-11185-x.

Prager, Sarah, Elizabeth Micks, and Vanessa K. Dalton, "Pregnancy Loss
    (Miscarriage): Terminology, Risk Factors, and Etiology," UpTo-
    Date, last updated September 24, 20021, https://www.uptodate.
    com/contents/pregnancy-loss-miscarriage-terminology-risk-
    factors-and-etiology.

"Preterm Birth," Centers for Disease Control and Prevention, last modi-
    fied November 1, 2021, https://www.cdc.gov/reproductive
    health/maternalinfanthealth/pretermbirth.htm.

Pruitt, Shannon M., Donna L. Hoyert, Kayla N. Anderson, Joyce Martin, Lisa Waddell, Charles Duke, Margaret A. Honein, and Jennita Reefhuis, "Racial and Ethnic Disparities in Fetal Deaths— United States, 2015–2017," *Morbidity and Mortality Weekly Report Weekly* 69, no. 37 (September 18, 2020): 1277–1282. https://www.cdc.gov/mmwr/volumes/69/wr/mm6937a1.htm.

Qu, Fan, Yan Wu, Yu-Hang Zhu, John Barry, Tao Ding, Gianluca Baio, Ruth Muscat, Brenda K. Todd, Fang-Fang Wang, and Paul J. Hardiman, "The Association between Psychological Stress and Miscarriage: A Systematic Review and Meta-Analysis," *Scientific Reports* 7 (2017): art. 1731. http://doi.org/10.1038/s41598-017-01792-3.

Quenby, Siobhan, Ioannis D. Gallos, Rima K. Dhillon-Smith, Marcelina Podesek, Mary D. Stephenson, Joanne Fisher, Jan J. Brosens, Jane Brewin, Rosanna Ramhorst, Emma S. Lucas, Rajiv C. McCoy, Robert Anderson, Shahd Daher, Lesley Regan, Maya Al-Memar, Tom Bourne, David A MacIntyre, Raj Rai, Ole B. Christiansen, Mayumi Sugiura-Ogasawara, Joshua Odendaal, Adam J. Devall, Phillip R. Bennett, Stavros Petrou, Arri Coomarasamy, "Miscarriage Matters: The Epidemiological, Physical, Psychological, and Economic Costs of Early Pregnancy Loss," *Lancet*, 397, no. 10285 (May 2021):1658–1667. https://doi.org/10.1016/S0140-6736(21)00682-6.

Quick Facts: Colorado, July 1, 2021, United States Census Bureau, https://www.census.gov/quickfacts/CO#qf-headnote-a.

Rainford, Monique, "America's Maternal Nightmare," Filmed September 27, 2018, TED video, https://www.ted.com/talks/monique_rainford_america_s_maternal_nightmare.

Raley, R. Kelly, Megan M. Sweeney, and Danielle Wondra, "The Growing Racial and Ethnic Divide in U.S. Marriage Patterns," *Future Child* 25, no. 2 (Fall 2015): 89–109. https://doi.org/10.1353/foc.2015.0014.

Ranji, Usha, Ivette Gomez, and Alina Salganicoff, "Expanding Postpartum Medicaid Coverage," Women's Health Policy, Kaiser Family Foundation, March 9, 2021, https://www.kff.org/womens-health-policy/issue-brief/expanding-postpartum-medicaid-coverage/.

Rasmussen, Morten, Mitsu Reddy, Rory Nolan, Joan Camunas-Soler, Arkady Khodursky, Nikolai M. Scheller, David E. Cantonwine, Line Engelbrechtsen, Jia Dai Mi, Arup Dutta, Tiffany Brundage, Farooq Siddiqui, Mainou Thao, Elaine P. S. Gee, Johnny La, Courtney Baruch-Gravett, Mark K. Santillan, Saikat Deb, Shaali M. Ame, Said M. Ali, Melanie Adkins, Mark A. DePristo, Manfred Lee, Eugeni Namsaraev, Dorte Jensen Gybel-Brask, Lillian Skibsted, James A. Litch, Donna A. Santillan, Sunil Sazawal, Rachel M. Tribe, James M. Roberts, Maneesh Jain, Estrid Høgdall, Claudia Holzman, Stephen R. Quake, Michal A. Elovitz, and Thomas F. McElrath, "RNA Profiles Reveal Signatures of Future Health and Disease in Pregnancy," *Nature*, no. 601 (2022): 422–427. https://doi.org/10.1038/s41586-021-04249-w.

Rauh-Hain, Jose A., Sarosh Rana, Hector Tamez, Alice Wang, Bruce Cohen, Allison Cohen, Florence Brown, Jeffrey L. Ecker, S. Ananth Karumanchi, and Ravi Thadhani, "Risk for Developing Gestational Diabetes in Women with Twin Pregnancies," *Journal of Maternal Fetal-Neonatal Medicine* 22, no. 4 (2009): 293–299. http://doi.org/10.1080/14767050802663194.

Rayburn, William F., Imam M. Xierali, Laura Castillo-Page, and Marc A. Nivet, "Racial and Ethnic Differences Between Obstetrician-Gynecologists and Other Adult Medical Specialists," *Obstetrics & Gynecology* 127, no. 1 (January 2016): 148–152. http://doi.org/10.1097/AOG.0000000000001184.

Razzaghi, Hilda, Mehreen Meghani, Cassandra Pingali, Bradley Crane, Allison Naleway, Eric Weintraub, Tat'Yana A. Kenigsberg, Mark J. Lamias, Stephanie A. Irving, Tia L. Kauffman, Kimberly K. Vesco, Matthew F. Daley, Malini DeSilva, James Donahue, Darios Getahun, Sungching Glenn, Simon J. Hambidge, MD, Lisa Jackson, Heather S. Lipkind, Jennifer Nelson, Ousseny Zerbo, Titilope Oduyebo, James A. Singleton, and Suchita A. Patel, "COVID-19 Vaccination Coverage Among Pregnant Women During Pregnancy—Eight Integrated Health Care Organizations, United States, December 14, 2020–May 8, 2021," *Morbidity and Mortality Weekly Report* 70, no. 24 (June 18, 2021): 895–899. https://www.cdc.gov/mmwr/volumes/70/wr/mm7024e2.htm.

Report from Maternal Mortality Review Committees: A View into Their Critical Role, 2017, https://reviewtoaction.org/national-resource/report-mmrcs-view-their-critical-role.

The Resident, Season 2 episode 20, "If Not Now When," directed by Rob Corn, featuring Malcome Jamal-Warner, Manish Dayal, and Shaunette Renee Wilson, aired April 15, 2019, on Fox.

Rivero, Enrique, "Proportion of Black Physicians in U.S. Has Changed Little in 120 Years, UCLA Research Finds," UCLA Newsroom, April 19, 2021, https://newsroom.ucla.edu/releases/proportion-black-physicians-little-change.

Roberts, Sam, "Yvette Fay Francis-McBarnette, a Pioneer in Treating Sickle Cell Anemia, Dies at 89," *New York Times*, April 7, 2016, https://www.nytimes.com/2016/04/08/nyregion/yvette-fay-francis-mcbarnette-a-pioneer-in-treating-sickle-cell-anemia-dies-at-89.html.

Roediger, David R., "Historical Foundations of Race," National Museum of African American History and Culture, accessed April 17, 2022, https://nmaahc.si.edu/learn/talking-about-race/topics/historical-foundations-race.

Rose, David, "A History of the March of Dimes," March of Dimes, August 26, 2010, https://www.marchofdimes.org/mission/a-history-of-the-march-of-dimes.aspx.

Rosenstein, Melissa G., Shen-Chih Chang, Christa Sakowski, Cathie Markow, Stephanie Teleki, Lance Lang, Julia Logan, Valerie Cape, and Elliott K. Main, "Hospital Quality Improvement Interventions, Statewide Policy Initiatives, and Rates of Cesarean Delivery for Nulliparous, Term, Singleton, Vertex Births in California," *JAMA* 325, no. 16 (2021): 1631–1639. https://doi.org/10.1001/jama.2021.3816.

Ruggles, Steven, "The Origins of African-American Family Structure," *American Sociological Review* 59 (February 1994): 136–151. https://users.pop.umn.edu/~ruggles/Articles/Af-Am-fam.pdf.

Sabin, Janice A., Brian A. Nosek, Anthony G. Greenwald, and Frederick P. Rivara, "Physicians' Implicit and Explicit Attitudes About Race by MD Race, Ethnicity, and Gender," *Journal of Health Care for the Poor and Underserved* 20, no. 3 (August 2009): 896–913. https://doi.org/10.1353/hpu.0.0185.

Sachs, Benjamin P., Cindy Kobelin, Mary Ames Castro, and Fredric Frigoletto, "The Risks of Lowering the Cesarean-Delivery Rate," *New England Journal of Medicine*, no. 340 (January 1999): 54–57. https://doi.org/10.1056/NEJM199901073400112.

Sacks, Vanessa, and David Murphey, "The Prevalence of Adverse Childhood Experiences, Nationally, by State, and by Race or Ethnicity," Child Trends, February 12, 2018, https://www.childtrends.org/publications/prevalence-adverse-childhood-experiences-nationally-state-race-ethnicity.

SACRED Birth during COVID19, University of California San Francisco, accessed June 6, 2022, https://sacredbirth.ucsf.edu/.

"Safe Prevention of the Primary Cesarean Delivery," *Obstetrics Care Consensus*, no. 1, March 2014, https://www.acog.org/clinical/clinical-guidance/obstetric-care-consensus/articles/2014/03/safe-prevention-of-the-primary-Cesarean-delivery.

Saftlas, Audrey F., Lisa M. Koonin, and Hani K. Atrash, "Racial Disparity in Pregnancy-Related Mortality Associated with Livebirth: Can Established Risk Factors Explain It?," *American Journal of Epidemiology* 152, no. 5 (September 2000): 413–419. https://doi.org/10.1093/aje/152.5.413.

Salameh, Taghreed N., Lynne A. Hall, Timothy N. Crawford, Ruth R. Staten, and Martin T. Hall, "Racial/Ethnic Differences in Mental Health Treatment among a National Sample of Pregnant Women with Mental Health and/or Substance Use Disorders in the United States," *Journal of Psychosomatic Research*, no. 121 (June 2019): 74–80. https://doi.org/10.1016/j.jpsychores.2019.03.015.

Sandall, Jane, Hora Soltani, Simon Gates, Andrew Shennan, and Declan Devane, "Midwife-led Continuity Models Versus Other Models of Care for Childbearing Women," *Cochrane Database of Systematic Reviews*, no. 4 (April 2016), https://doi.org/10.1002/14651858.CD004667.pub5.

Say, Lale, Doris Chou, Alison Gemmill, Özge Tunçalp, Ann-Beth Moller, Jane Daniels, A. Metin Gülmezoglu, Marleen Temmerman, Leontine Alkema, "Global Causes of Maternal Death: A WHO Systematic Analysis," *Lancet* 2, no. 6 (June 2014): E323, https://doi.org/10.1016/S2214-109X(14)70227-X.

Schernhammer, Eva S., and Graham A. Colditz, "Suicide Rates among Physicians: A Quantitative and Gender Assessment (Meta-analysis)," *American Journal of Psychiatry* 161, no. 12 (December 2004): 2295–2302. https://doi.org/10.1176/appi. ajp.161.12.2295.

Schumacher, Joel, dir., *A Time to Kill* (Warner Brothers, 1996).

Scommegna, Paola, "High Premature Birth Rates Among U.S. Black Women May Reflect the Stress of Racism and Health and Economic Factors," Population Reference Bureau, January 21, 2021, https://www.prb.org/resources/high-premature-birth-rates-among-u-s-black-women-may-reflect-the-stress-of-racism-and-health-and-economic-factors/.

Scott, Karen A., MD, MPH, FACOG, Founding CEO and Owner, personal website, Birthing Cultural Rigor, LLC, Public Health Institute, accessed June 5, 2022, https://www.phi.org/experts/karen-a-scott/.

Seaton, E. K., C. H. Caldwell, R. M. Sellers, and J. S. Jackson, "The Prevalence of Perceived Discrimination among African American and Caribbean Black Youth," *Developmental Psychology* 44, no. 5 (2008): 1288–1297. https://doi.org/10.1037/a0012747.

Seeman, Teresa E., Bruce S. McEwen, John W. Rowe, and Burton H. Singer, "Allostatic Load as a Marker of Cumulative Biological Risk: MacArthur Studies of Successful Aging," *PNAS* 98, no. 8 (April 2001): 4770–4775. https://doi.org/10.1073/pnas.081072698.

Shah, Neel, MD, MPP, Assistant Professor, personal website, Harvard Medical School, accessed June 6, 2022, https://scholar.harvard.edu/shah/home.

Shah, Prakesh S., Jamie Zao, and Samana Ali, "Maternal Marital Status and Birth Outcomes: A Systematic Review and Meta-analyses," *Maternal and Child Health Journal* 15, no. 7 (2011): 1097–1109. https://doi.org/10.1007/s10995-010-0654-z.

Shammas, Masood A., "Telomeres, Lifestyle, Cancer, and Aging," *Current Opinion in Clinical Nutrition & Metabolic Care* 14, no. 1 (January 2011): 28–34. https://doi.org/10.1097/MCO.0b013e32834121b1.

"Sickle Cell Disease (SCD)," Centers for Disease Control and Prevention, last updated May 25, 2022, https://www.cdc.gov/ncbddd/sicklecell/index.html.

Simms, Tanya M., Carol E. Rodriguez, Rosa Rodriguez, and Rene J. Herrera, "The Genetic Structure of Populations from Haiti and Jamaica Reflect Divergent Demographic Histories," *American Journal of Physical Anthropology* 142, no. 1 (2010): 49–66. https://doi.org/10.1002/ajpa.21194.

Singh, Gopal K., "Trends and Social Inequalities in Maternal Mortality in the United States, 1969–2018," *International Journal of Maternal and Child Health and AIDS* 10, no. 1 (2021): 29–42. https://doi.org/10.21106/ijma.444.

Siu, Albert L., and US Preventive Services Task Force (USPSTF), "Screening for Depression in Adults: US Preventive Services Task Force Recommendation Statement," *JAMA* 315, no. 4 (January 2016): 380–387. https://doi.org/10.1001/jama.2015.18392.

Smith, Susan E., Nina Sivertsen, Lauren Lines, and Anita De Bellis, "Decision Making in Vaccine Hesitant Parents and Pregnant Women—An Integrative Review," *International Journal of Nursing Studies Advances* 4 (December 2022). https://doi.org/10.1016/j.ijnsa.2022.100062.

"Smoking During Pregnancy," Centers for Disease Control and Prevention, last modified April 28, 2020, https://www.cdc.gov/tobacco/basic_information/health_effects/pregnancy/index.htm.

Snyder, Alison, "Yvette Fay Francis-McBarnette," *Lancet* 387, no. 10031 (May 7, 2016): 1092, https://doi.org/10.1016/S0140-6736(16)30411-1.

"Society for Maternal-Fetal Medicine (SMFM) Statement: SARS-CoV-2 Vaccination in Pregnancy," Society for Maternal Fetal Medicine, December 1, 2020, https://s3.amazonaws.com/cdn.smfm.org/media/2591/SMFM_Vaccine_Statement_12-1-20_(final).pdf.

Solomon, Judith, "Closing the Coverage Gap Would Improve Black Maternal Health," Center on Budget and Policy Priorities, July 26, 2021, https://www.cbpp.org/research/health/closing-the-coverage-gap-would-improve-black-maternal-health.

Souter, Vivienne, Elizabeth Nethery, Mary Lou Kopas, Hannah Wurz, Kristin Sitcov, and Aaron B. Caughey, "Comparison of

Midwifery and Obstetric Care in Low-Risk Hospital Births," *Obstetrics & Gynecology* 134, no. 5 (November 2019): 1056– 1065. https://doi.org/10.1097/AOG.0000000000003521.

Spong, C. Y., M. Beall, D. Rodrigues, and M. G. Ross, "An Objective Definition of Shoulder Dystocia: Prolonged Head-to-Body Delivery Intervals and/or the Use of Ancillary Obstetric Maneuvers," *Obstetrics & Gynecology* 86, no. 3 (1995): 433–436. https://doi.org/10.1016/0029-7844(95)00188-W.

Stephen, Elizabeth Hervey, and Anjani Chandra, "Declining Estimates of Infertility in the United States: 1982–2002," *Fertility and Sterility* 86, no. 3 (2006): 516–523, https://doi.org/10.1016/j.fertnstert.2006.02.129.

Stern, Alexandra Minna, "Forced Sterilization Policies in the US Targeted Minorities and Those with Disabilities—and Lasted Into the 21st Century," University of Michigan Institute for Healthcare and Policy and Innovation News, September 23, 2020, https://ihpi.umich.edu/news/forced-sterilization-policies-us-targeted-minorities-and-those-disabilities-and-lasted-21st.

———, "That Time the United States Sterilized 60,000 of Its Citizens," *Huffpost*, January 7, 2016, https://www.huffpost.com/entry/sterilization-united-states_n_568f35f2e4b0c8beacf68713.

Stewart, Elizabeth A., Wanda K. Nicholson, Linda Bradley, and Bijan J. Borah, "The Burden of Uterine Fibroids for African-American Women: Results of a National Survey," *Journal of Women's Health* 22, no. 10 (October 2013): 807–816. http://doi.org/10.1089/jwh.2013.4334.

"Sudden Unexpected Infant Death and Sudden Infant Death Syndrome, Centers for Disease Control and Prevention, last updated June 21, 2022, https://www.cdc.gov/sids/data.htm.

Swartz, Mark, "The Bridgeport Baby Bundle: Thinking in Systems, not Programs," Early Learning Nation, April 15, 2021, https://earlylearningnation.com/2021/04/the-bridgeport-baby-bundle-thinking-in-systems-not-programs/.

Tanabe, Kawai O., and Fern R. Hauck, "A United States Perspective," in *SIDS Sudden Infant and Early Childhood Death: The Past, the Present and the Future*, ed. Jhodie R. Duncan and Roger W.

Byard (Adelaide: University of Adelaide Press, 2018), https://
www.ncbi.nlm.nih.gov/books/NBK513376/.

Tessum, Christopher W., David A. Paolella, Sarah E. Chambliss, Joshua
S. Apte, Jason D. Hill, and Julian D. Marshall, "PM2.5 Polluters
Disproportionately and Systemically Affect People of Color
in the United States," *Science Advances* 7, no. 18 (April 2021),
http://doi.org/10.1126/sciadv.abf4491.

Thornburg, Kent L., Jackilen Shannon, Philippe Thuillier, and Mitchell
S. Turker, "In Utero Life and Epigenetic Predisposition for
Disease," *Advances in Genetics*, no. 71 (2010): 57–78. https://doi.
org/10.1016/B978-0-12-380864-6.00003-1.

Tikkanen, Roosa, Munira Z. Gunja, Molly FitzGerald, and Laurie Zeph-
yrin, "Maternal Mortality and Maternity Care in the United States
Compared to 10 Other Developed Countries," Commonwealth
Fund, November 18, 2020, https://www.commonwealthfund
.org/publications/issue-briefs/2020/nov/maternal-mortality
-maternity-care-us-compared-10-countries.

Troja, Achim, Ahmed Abdou, Christiane Rapp, Swantje Wienand,
Eduard Malik, and Hans-Rudolf Raaba, "Management of Spontaneous Hepatic Rupture on Top of HELLP Syndrome: Case
Report and Review of the Literature," *Viszeralmedizin* 31, no. 3
(2015): 205–208. https://doi.org/10.1159/000376601.

"Twin Birth Rates in the United States between 1980 and 2019, by
Ethnicity," statista, February 2022, https://www.statista.com/
statistics/244913/twin-birth-rates-in-the-united-states-by-
ethnicity/.

"Understanding Changes in Life Expectancy," Cystic Fibrosis Foundation, accessed May 9, 2022, https://www.cff.org/managing-cf/
understanding-changes-life-expectancy.

United States Department of Health and Human Services, Health
Resources and Services Administration, National Center for
Health Workforce Analysis, *Projections of Supply and Demand
for Women's Health Service Providers: 2018–2030*, March
2021, https://bhw.hrsa.gov/sites/default/files/bureau-health-
workforce/data-research/projections-supply-demand-2018-
2030.pdf.

US Preventive Services Task Force, "Aspirin Use to Prevent Preeclampsia and Related Morbidity and Mortality: US Preventive Services Task Force Recommendation Statement," *JAMA* 326, no. 12 (2021): 1186–1191. https://doi.org/10.1001/jama.2021.14781.

"U.S.-born Black Women at Higher Risk of Preeclampsia than Black Immigrants," American Heart Association Newsroom, November 9, 2020, https://newsroom.heart.org/news/u-s-born-black-women-at-higher-risk-of-preeclampsia-than-black-immigrants.

"Vaginal Birth after Cesarean Delivery," *ACOG Practice Bulletin*, no. 205 (February 2019), https://www.acog.org/clinical/clinical-guidance/practice-bulletin/articles/2019/02/vaginal-birth-after-Cesarean-delivery.

van Ryn, Michelle, and Steven S. Fu, "Paved with Good Intentions: Do Public Health and Human Service Providers Contribute to Racial/Ethnic Disparities in Health?," *American Journal of Public Health* 93, no. 2 (February 2003): 248–255. https://doi.org/10.2105/AJPH.93.2.248.

VanGompel, Emily White, Jin-Shei Lai, Dána-Ain Davis, Francesca Carlock, Tamentanefer L. Camara, Brianne Taylor, Chakiya Clary, Ashlee M. McCorkle-Jamieson, Safyer McKenzie-Sampson, Caryl Gay, Amanda Armijo, Lillie Lapeyrolerie, Lavisha Singh, and Karen A. Scott, "Psychometric Validation of a Patient-Reported Experience Measure of Obstetric Racism© (The PREM-OB Scale™ Suite)," *Birth* (March 17, 2022): 514–525. https://doi.org/10.1111/birt.12622.

Villarosa, Linda, "Why America's Black Mothers and Babies Are in a Life-or-Death Crisis," *New York Times*, April 11, 2018, https://www.nytimes.com/2018/04/11/magazine/black-mothers-babies-death-maternal-mortality.html.

———, *Under the Skin: The Hidden Toll of Racism on American Lives and the Health of Our Nation* (New York: Doubleday, 2022).

Volscho, Thomas W., "Sterilization Racism and Pan-ethnic Disparities of the Last Decade: The Continued Encroachment on Reproductive Rights," *Wicazo Sa Review: A Journal of Native American Studies*, 25, no. 1 (2010): 17–31. https://doi.org/10.1353/wic.0.0053.

Wade, Sabia C., (website), accessed June 5, 2022, https://www.sabi-awade.com.

Wallack, Lawrence, and Kent L. Thornburg, "Developmental Origins, Epigenetics, and Equity: Moving Upstream," *Maternal Child Health Journal* 20, no. 5 (May 2016): 935–940. https://doi.org/10.1007/s10995-016-1970-8.

Wastnedge, Elizabeth, Donald Waters, Sarah R. Murray, Brian McGowan, Effie Chipeta, Alinane Linda Nyondo-Mipando, Luis Gadama, Gladys Gadama, Martha Masamba, Monica Malata, Frank Taulo, Queen Dube, Kondwani Kawaza, Patricia Munthali Khomani, Sonia Whyte, Mia Crampin, Bridget Freyne, Jane E. Norman, and Rebecca M. Reynolds, "Interventions to Reduce Preterm Birth and Stillbirth, and Improve Outcomes for Babies Born Preterm in Low- and Middle-Income Countries: A Systematic Review," *Journal of Global Health*, no. 1 (2021), https://jogh.org/2021/jogh-11-04050.

Wellons, Melissa F., Cora E. Lewis, Stephen M. Schwartz, Erica P. Gunderson, Pamela J. Schreiner, Barbara Sternfeld, Josh Richman, Cynthia K. Sites, and David S. Siscovick, "Racial Differences in Self-Reported Infertility and Risk Factors for Infertility in a Cohort of Black and White Women: The CARDIA Women's Study," *Fertility and Sterility* 90, no. 5 (2008): 1640–1648. https://doi.org/10.1016/j.fertnstert.2007.09.056.

Wesselink, Amelia K., Lynn Rosenberg, Lauren A. Wise, Michael Jerrett, Patricia F. Coogan, "A Prospective Cohort Study of Ambient Air Pollution Exposure and Risk of Uterine Leiomyomata," *Human Reproduction* 36, no. 8 (August 2021): 2321–2330. https://doi.org/10.1093/humrep/deab095.

"What is Epigenetics?," Centers for Disease Control and Prevention, last updated May 18, 2022, https://www.cdc.gov/genomics/disease/epigenetics.htm.

"What is Stillbirth?," Centers for Disease Control and Prevention, last modified November 16, 2020, https://www.cdc.gov/ncbddd/stillbirth/facts.html.

White, Gillian B., "Black Workers Really Do Need to Be Twice as Good," *Atlantic*, October 7, 2015, https://www.theatlantic.com

/business/archive/2015/10/why-black-workers-really-do-need-to-be-twice-as-good/409276/.

White, Taneasha, and Jacquelyn Johnson, "Racism in Mental Health Care: Where Are We Now?," PsychCentral, April 4, 2022, https://psychcentral.com/health/racism-in-mental-health-care.

"What We Do," National Birth Equity Collaborative, accessed June 5, 2022, https://birthequity.org/what-we-do/.

"Who We Are," Irth (Birth Without Bias) App, accessed June 3, 2022, https://irthapp.com/who-we-are/.

"Who We Are," March of Dimes, accessed June 11, 2022, https://www.marchofdimes.org/mission/who-we-are.aspx.

"Why Ob-Gyns Are Burning Out," American College of Obstetricians and Gynecologists, October 28, 2019, https://www.acog.org/news/news-articles/2019/10/why-ob-gyns-are-burning-out.

Williams, Heather Andrea, "How Slavery Affected African American Families," Freedom's Story, TeacherServe. National Humanities Center, accessed April 24, 2022, http://nationalhumanities center.org/tserve/freedom/1609-1865/essays/aafamilies.htm.

Williams, Oneeka, *Not Today Negativity!* (Newtonville, MA: Dr. Dee Dee Dynamo Books 2021).

Williams, Serena, "How Serena Williams Saved Her Own Life," *Elle*, April 25, 2022, https://www.elle.com/life-love/a39586444/how-serena-williams-saved-her-own-life/S.

Willinger, Marian, Chia-Wen Ko, and Uma M. Reddy, "Racial Disparities in Stillbirth Risk Across Gestation in the United States," *American Journal of Obstetrics and Gynecology* 201, no. 5 (November 2009): 469.e1. https://doi.org/10.1016%2Fj.ajog.2009.06.057.

Yamamoto, A., M.C. McCormick, and H.H. Burris, "Disparities in Antidepressant Use in Pregnancy," *Journal of Perinatology* 35 (2015): 246–251. https://doi.org/10.1038/jp.2014.197.

Yang, Yawei J., Elisabeth A. Murphy, Sunidhi Singh, Ashley C. Sukhu, Isabel Wolfe, Sanjana Adurty, Dorothy Eng, Jim Yee, Iman Mohammed, Zhen Zhao, Laura E. Riley, and Malavika Prabhu, "Association of Gestational Age at Coronavirus Disease 2019 (COVID-19) Vaccination, History of Severe Acute Respiratory Syndrome Coronavirus 2 (SARS-CoV-2) Infection, and a Vaccine Booster Dose with Maternal and Umbilical

Cord Antibody Levels at Delivery," *Obstetrics & Gynecology* 139, no. 3 (March 2022): 373–380. https://doi.org/10.1097/ AOG.0000000000004693.

Yao, Ruofan, Cande V. Ananth, Bo Y. Park, Leanne Pereira, and Lauren A. Plante, "Obesity and the Risk of Stillbirth: A Population-Based Cohort Study," *American Journal of Obstetrics and Gyne- cology* 210, no. 5 (May 2014): 457.e1. https://doi.org/10.1016/j. ajog.2014.01.044.

Zambrano, Laura D., Sascha Ellington, Penelope Strid, Romeo R. Galang, Titilope Oduyebo, Van T. Tong, Kate R. Wood- worth, John F. Nahabedian III, Eduardo Azziz-Baumgartner, Suzanne M. Gilboa, and Dana Meaney-Delman, "Update: Characteristics of Symptomatic Women of Reproductive Age with Laboratory-Confirmed SARS-CoV-2 Infection by Preg- nancy Status—United States, January 22–October 3, 2020," *Morbidity and Mortality Weekly Report* 69, no. 44 (November 6, 2020): 1641–1641. https://www.cdc.gov/mmwr/volumes/69/ wr/mm6944e3.htm.